Vegan

Vegan Diet for Easy Weight Loss and Healthy Living through Natural Foods

Brian Adams

Brian Adams

Disclaimer Notice:

Please note the information contained within this document is for educational and entertainment purposes only. Every attempt has been made to provide accurate, up to date and reliable complete information. No warranties of any kind are expressed or implied. Readers acknowledge that the author is not engaging in the rendering of legal, financial, medical or professional advice.

By reading this document, the reader agrees that under no circumstances are we responsible for any losses, direct or indirect, which are incurred as a result of the use of information contained within this document, including, but not limited to, — errors, omissions, or inaccuracies.

Table of Contents

Brian Adams

Introduction

Gone are the days when we had enough time for everything, back when the world was not so competitive. In this fast pacing world, we compromise the time spent on anything that is not work. Strained relationships and unhealthy eating habits are the two major offshoots of this gamble.

With the less amount of time that we have at our disposal and the large number of activities we need to do in that less amount of time, it is often that our person to person relationships and our health that take a backseat. With the ever increasing strain on us, we always try to take a quicker and easier way out; returning calls with texts, and using a "Skype dates" to compensate for our lack of person to person interaction.

With very less time available to cook, we often end up taking the easy route of processed foods and fast foods. What is the price that we pay for these quick fix solutions? Obesity, being the primary consequence of unhealthy dietary habits, has been the cause for many health related issues. To make good the extra pounds, we are often in the lookout for that perfect diet.

But, a lot of diets place a lot of restrictions on us, calling for fancy foods and ingredients that we need to Google to even know what they look like! These ingredients are often available only at specialty stores and cost a bomb! Like mentioned earlier, we do not even have time to cook, how will we find the time to go off on a treasure hunt to faraway stores, looking for the ingredients demanded by the fancy diet?

Allow us to introduce you to the Vegan diet, which is a failsafe way to not only knock those extra pounds but also to welcome a healthy lifestyle. You will realize that there is a tremendous shift in how you regard animals once you turn a Vegan and that insight could be a real eye-opener.

Though the vegan diet is quite popular and is often termed to be a "fad", a lot of studies have shown and proven that it does actually work in helping people lose those much needed pounds. But, despite its popularity, the knowledge of most people regarding the diet is vague at its best. Most people know the general instructions of the diet (i.e., avoid products derived from animals); most people are unaware of the crux!

We are sure that your head must be swarming with questions like- "What goes into a vegan diet?" "What are its benefits?" "How is it any different and effective?" Well, you have come to the right place to know all that you need to know about the vegan diet.

In the first chapter of this book, we have given an overview of Veganism and the reasons for resorting to it. In the second chapter you will find an interesting read on the history of veganism and its branching out from vegetarianism. This chapter also contains the ethics veganism is based upon. In the third and fourth chapters, we have highlighted the many benefits of adopting the vegan diet. We have elucidated the tips to adopt this diet with ease in the fifth chapter. The fifth chapter also discusses some commonly asked nutritional health questions about adoption of a vegan diet. It helps dispel some myths and increases awareness for some much needed nutritional cornerstones. The sixth chapter contains a list of foods that you can consume, the foods that you need to avoid and the substitutes you can use for the non-vegan food items. The seventh chapter will outline a few simple sample menus, highlighting how you should be combining nutrition in all three meals. It also gives you a number of easy exercises that will help you shed off the pounds in no time.

The last six chapters are the most interesting of the lot, as we bring to you exciting and easy to follow recipes that are quick to make and will get you on the highway to better health in no time at all!

The eighth chapter contains breakfast recipes that will help you get an exciting, healthy and delicious start to your day. The ninth chapter contains delicious soup recipes that will set the tone for your meal, and sometimes, be a meal by themselves.

The tenth chapter contains recipes for moth watering main dishes, while the eleventh chapter contains side dishes to accompany the delectable main dishes. The twelfth chapter contains a number of unique salad recipes, highlighting the fact that salads are not always raw rabbit food. They are delectable and often main dishes themselves.

The last chapter is the most exciting as it contains recipes for desserts! Yes, desserts on a diet to lose weight! These tempting and heavenly desserts are extremely healthy and won't mess up your diet in any way; rather they will supplement your diet.

We hope you find the answers to all your questions in this book! Thank you for purchasing this book and we hope the content is helpful!

Chapter 1: Veganism – An Overview

It is important that we understand what goes into a Vegan diet to understand how beneficial it is. The right term to use here would be to understand what does not go into a Vegan diet. In this chapter, we have given an overview of Veganism and what it is all about.

Who is a Vegan?

Vegans do not include meat products, milk, dairy and egg products in their diet. They also abstain from using animal products like leather, hide etc.

Vegans are often confused with vegetarians and that is the biggest misconception. Veganism is a part of vegetarianism albeit a stricter one. Let us understand the kinds of vegetarians first to understand more about veganism.

Vegetarians are classified into four categories based on the type of foods consumed. They are as follows:

> ➤ Lacto- Ovo Vegetarian: Does not include fowl, fish or meat, but includes egg and dairy products.
> ➤ Ovo Vegetarian: Does not include dairy products, fish, fowl and meat, but includes egg products.
> ➤ Lacto Vegetarian: Does not include egg products, fish, fowl and meat, but includes dairy products.
> ➤ Vegan: Does not include dairy products, fish, fowl, meat, egg products and honey. They abstain from using animal products such as leather, silk etc.

Why Veganism?

Veganism is generally adopted for several reasons. The reasons why people turn vegan are as follows:

Environment:

People resort to veganism because of the hazards associated with livestock farming. We seldom realize the impacts of livestock farming on our environment. Only healthy livestock is sold as meat. To ensure that the livestock is healthy, they are fed fodder of high quality. This increases the demand for crops and fodder, thereby increasing the demand for food production. This in turn increases the pressure on the soil and leads to soil erosion. It has also been significantly contributing towards global warming and resultantly food security concerns have increased. The overall impact on the environment tends to branch out in consumption of already limited fresh water resources. It also requires an increased amount of land resource thus heightening the issue of encroachment on forests. Deforestation is therefore another offshoot of this issue. The increased pressure on food production can be reduced considerably if there is a decline in livestock farming. Increased dependence on plant-based diets can reduce this impact significantly as well as creating a more sustainable food source over the long run. To ensure that the balance in the ecosystem is restored, people opt for veganism.

Animal rights:

Vegetarianism strives to address animal rights issues. However, Vegans regard animal rights in a more serious light than the other kinds of vegetarians.

Apart from shunning any kind of meat from their diets, Vegans also eliminate honey, dairy products and egg products, even though these do not harm animals. You might wonder why

Vegans eliminate these food items, even though they do not harm animals. This mainly flows from their belief that animals have the rights of existence and survival without the interference of mankind. They believe that man has no right to steal the milk, honey and eggs from animals. Apart from these, they also refrain from using animal products such as wool, leather, silk etc. Harvesting wool may not harm animals, but the animals bred for wool are kept in terrible conditions and vegans feel this is ethically incorrect. These initial assertions that motivate the diet change can often be reinforced and augmented through various other motivations over time. While an individual might begin with one preference, the beliefs could strengthen over time with increased restriction on one's diet.

Health:

Choosing to be a vegan has a lot of health benefits. Apart from the celebrated benefit of weight reduction, Vegan diet has other health benefits as well. Health concerns have also been a key instigator in adoption of a vegan diet. Since veganism holds multiple health benefits it is often considered a boon in relation to the various ethical stances committed vegans hold dear. Health benefits of veganism are numerous and are beneficial to a number of issues.

The risk of developing rheumatoid arthritis, diabetes, hypertension, various cardiovascular diseases and diabetes in increased because of the consumption of dairy products and meat. The risks of the abovementioned diseases are eliminated when one adopts the Vegan diet. People who generally stand the chance of contracting chronic cardiac diseases shift to Vegan diet to reduce the risk.

The major constituents of the Vegan diet include fruits, legumes, vegetables and whole grains. These have no cholesterol and have low or no fat content. These are also rich in anti-oxidants thereby helping you to remain active throughout the day.

Brian Adams

Chapter 2: History of Veganism

Veganism is a practice that consists of completely refraining from using animal products. Veganism is an extreme form of vegetarianism and involves complete abstinence from animal products whether edible or inedible. Vegans are often prompted by a set of beliefs that includes rejection of the commodity status of animals. The idea progresses in light of a lifestyle that does not depend on the exploitation of animals.

This idea takes stock of various cultural preferences and includes ideals found in the ancient East Mediterranean and Indian societies. The practice of vegetarianism can also be traced back to 6th Century BCE where the renowned Greek philosopher and mathematician Pythagoras was in favor of benevolence towards animals. In addition to Pythagoras, philosophers like Theophrastus and Empedocles were vegetarians, in addition to Ovid, Plutarch, Plotinus, Porphyry and Seneca the Younger. The focus on such a lifestyle came from the various philosophical beliefs held and developed by these illustrious men of their age. The arguments were based upon the transmigration of souls, benevolence towards animals and the overall issues of health and wellbeing. Hinduism, Jainism and Buddhism also follow similar doctrines of benevolence and transmigration of the soul. These religious beliefs have continued on to modern times and followers of such religions are mostly ardent believers and thus follow such dietary lifestyles. Vegetarianism is thus a very common occurrence in some societies.

Western societies have not seen a complete change of dietary choices and vegetarianism and consequently veganism have been part of upsurges as religious revivals and health fads. This however has always been substantiated by the health benefits that a well-balanced vegan diet has provided. Philosophers such as Jeremy Bentham, in the 18th Century postulated that animal suffering was as grave as human suffering. The Ephrata Cloister of Pennsylvania in 1732 promoted strict vegetarianism.

Vegetarianism found root in England and the United States of America in the 19th Century. William Lambe in 1815, a physician in London proposed a vegetarian diet in light of its health benefits and as a cure for cancer and asthma. The first vegetarian society came into being in 1847 in England, while in the United States Amos Bronson Alcott began two communities in Massachusetts in 1834 (Temple Schools) and 1844 (Fruitland's). Fruitland's in 1844 advocated the complete boycott of animal derived products. In 1838 James Pierrepont Greaves formed the Concordium as a vegan school and community in England. Alcott House is also responsible for the creation of the first vegan advocacy group in 1843. The Alcott House was a key character in creating the first vegetarian society in England in 1847. Three years post the formation of the British Vegetarian Society Reverend Sylvester Graham co-founded the American Vegetarian Society. He is also famous for the invention of Graham Crackers and was a Presbyterian Minister. He advocated a virtuous life which was based on principles of vegetarianism, temperance and abstinence as well as proper hygiene. His followers were known as the Grahamites followed these doctrines and could be considered amongst practicing vegetarians.

Vegans are differentiated from vegetarians, as they do not consume any product that is derived from animals. A British Woodworker coined the term "vegan" and secretary of the Leicester Vegetarian Society by the name of Donald Watson in order to differentiate between vegetarians that consumed dairy products like milk and milk products (butter, cheese etc.) and eggs and those who completely abstained. He created a newsletter, 'Vegan News' in November 1944 and defined the term vegan, as it is known now. Popular vegans of the time included George Bernard Shaw. The World Vegan Day is celebrated on 1st November in order to pay homage to the creation of the newsletter.

A collection of individuals came together in response to the newsletter forming the new Vegan Society in London. The venue for the first meeting was the Attic Club 144 High Holborn London. This initiated a movement that enabled veganism to develop a greater scope and various issues of ethical usage started coming to light. The movement took cause with not only the vegan dietary choices but also with the usage of products that were animal friendly. The society placed recommendations for practicing vegans in terms of what products they could use while practicing complete avoidance of animal derived substances. Rubin Abramowitz and Catherine Nimmo formed following Watson's footsteps the first Vegan Society in 1948 and later in 1960 Jay Dinshah formed the formal American Vegan Society. Dinshah linked the idea of veganism to that of 'non-harming' or 'ahimsa' that originates from Sanskrit. This belies a connection with the ancient Hindu religious practices of transmigration of the soul and ideas of non-harm towards animals.

Vegan literature started being developed including recipes such as the book "Vegan Recipes" by Fay K. Henderson and "Aids to a Vegan Diet" by Kathleen V. Mayo. Donald Watson in 1947 stated a clear distinction between vegetarianism and veganism through stating a clear intent of renouncing the exploitation of animals under any circumstance. Veganism can also be credited with founding Plantmilk Limited; the company was founded by the vice-president of the Vegan Society and aimed at exploring the potential of soymilk as a potential replacement for dairy milk. Founded in 1965, the company has been a huge success with around 2 million liters of plant milk sold to consumers in the UK in 2013.

Vegan was formally defined in 1962 in the Oxford Dictionary as

"A person who does not eat or use animal products"

And states

"A vegetarian is an individual that eats no milk, eggs, butter, or cheese."

This defining distinction is what states vegan as different from vegetarian. Thus following a vegan diet often means a complete commitment to utilize only plant sourced products.

Ethical and Environmental Veganism:

Ethical veganism stems from an opposition of speciesism; an idea that develops a hierarchy and value in lieu of the species membership. Protectionism and abolitionism are two branches of ethical veganism; protectionism aims at a greater focus on the ethical treatment and handling of animals whereas abolitionism seeks to end all kinds of human ownership of animals. It focuses on the idea of intrinsic moral values for non-humans and economic gains are not a strong enough reason for justification for utilizing animals as food. Animal suffering should thus be accounted for in all decisions regarding their utilization. Sensitivity to circumstances of use is often considered consequentialist and according to abolitionists, reneges on its own values as it allows for infractions. Ethical veganism holds the idea that once declared. It is essential that the individual realize the cost and consequence of utilization of "all" animal products. This focuses the individual to commit to the ideal and not just choose areas, which they may want to follow.

Environmental veganism focuses on the idea of conservationism and overall sustainability of environment in light of domestication and farming of animals. In order to develop long-term sustainability, environmental vegans consider a switch to a majorly plant based diet. On an estimate around 30% of the surface of the earth is devoted to the livestock sector and over the long term this has a significant impact on resources like air, land, soil and water. The overall impact of animal husbandry comes in the way of increased greenhouse emissions as well as the sheer number of livestock and fish required to fulfill the global needs. This has led to dangerous and potentially devastating effects on the natural order, through loss of habitat for wild animals and over-fishing in the deep seas. Animal waste also increases the amount of harmful gases in the atmosphere, with the livestock industry responsible for 9% of anthropogenic carbon dioxide emissions, 65% of nitrous oxide, 68% of ammonia and 37% of the methane released in a single year. The overall environmental damage is only rising in costs and in order to have a long-term sustainability in the world food supply environmental vegans consider moving towards a plant based diet to be a better solution.

Rise of Modern Veganism:

Modern veganism started with Donald Watson and his definition of vegan; but it was mainly considered directed towards food consumption and was considered a replacement of the lengthy term of 'non-dairy vegetarians'. The decisive change in dietary lifestyle is what initiated the vegan movement but it also encompassed the overall focus on the prevalence of animal based products that increased not only the consumption in food but became integral in industry. Increased consumption meant increased environmental impacts as explained above. Leslie J. Cross who saw the need for a proper definition in order to put forward the actual aim of the movement defined veganism in 1949. Leslie J. Cross defined it as "the principle of the emancipation of animals from exploitation by man". Man later elucidated this by man for food, commodities, work, hunting, vivisection, and by all other uses involving exploitation of animal life". The final form and definition of veganism was updated in 1979 when the New Vegan Society of Donald Watson became a charity. The Memorandum and Articles of Association defined it as

"A philosophy and way of living which seeks to exclude—as far as is possible and practicable—all forms of exploitation of, and cruelty to, animals for food, clothing or any other purpose; and by extension, promotes the development and use of animal-free alternatives for the benefit of humans, animals and the environment. In dietary terms it denotes the practice of dispensing with all products derived wholly or partly from animals."

Chapter 3: Health Benefits of a Vegan Diet

As mentioned in the previous chapter, the Vegan diet has multiple health benefits. We have highlighted the important health benefits that one can derive by resorting to Vegan diet in this chapter. Not only does vegan diet help in developing a diverse palate but it also helps in the long run to reduce the onset of various diseases and keeps the body healthy.

- **Cataracts:**

  Fruits and vegetables are important constituents of the Vegan diet. These fruits and vegetables are a rich source of healthy anti-oxidants. These anti-oxidants play an important role in eliminating the risk of contracting cataracts. Vegan diet is exceptionally rich in anti-oxidants as many foods in vegan diet contain the vitamins ACE that are exceptional sources of anti-oxidants and phytochemicals, thus preventing free-radical damage.

- **Macular degeneration:**

Macular degeneration, which is one of the potential risks associated with old age, can be kept at bay by consuming fresh vegetables like carrots, sweet potatoes, pumpkins and leafy greens and fruits.

- **Osteoporosis:**

The four important factors that contribute to bone heath are adequate intake of protein and calcium, low sodium intake and high potassium intake. One way to ensure that the body gets the right amount of these four nutrients is to follow the vegan diet. By following the vegan diet, you ensure that your body receives the four important nutrients, but without the added disadvantages of other harmful components like lead, mercury, saturated fats, etc., that your body receives when you consume a few varieties of meat. When the bone health is taken care of, you can be sure that osteoporosis is at bay.

- **Vitamin C intake:**

The Vegan diet is rich in Vitamin C. The health of the gums is dependent on the Vitamin C intake. Apart from that, the immune system is also boosted by the intake of Vitamin C.

- **Skin Care:**

The nuts and vegetables that form a part of the Vegan diet are rich in Vitamin A content. Vitamin A is an important factor that promotes healthier skin. The vitamin A, vitamin C and vitamin E are all crucial in this respect as they provide the body with adequate anti-oxidants and thus reduce the damage on a cellular level. This increases the longevity of healthy cells and thus makes the skin retain its health and youthfulness for longer.

- **Water Content:**

Consumption of fresh fruits and vegetables ensures that the water content in the body is maintained. Potassium is essential in maintaining the balance of water in the body and aids in kidney function thus balancing and aiding the removal of toxins like excess sodium. Excessive sodium in the body can lead to water retention and a healthy body is dependent upon adequate balance of water.

- **Body Mass Index:**

As mentioned before, the Vegan diet has low or no fat and no cholesterol. Hence, the vegan diet helps in the reduction of weight and lowers the BMI of the individual. It is a well-known fact that people who follow the vegan diet have lower body mass indices. It is also rich in both soluble and insoluble fiber and aids in healthy bowels and digestion. Effective digestion also aids in keeping weight within healthy limits. A lower body mass index is indicative of a lower quantity of fat in the body, including and especially the harmful fat that surrounds internal organs and cannot be gauged by simple methods of weighing oneself. Even when individuals do not seem overweight or obese physically, this fat can be present and the best way to rid oneself of it is through a balanced diet that is low in saturated fat.

- **Weight Loss:**

By focusing on a vegan menu, it is often easier to eliminate excessively fatty substances from ones diet. Vegan diet is also naturally in low in bad fats and is therefore easier to follow while attempting weight loss. Most vegan foods do not need to be restricted in portioning due to their low calorie and fat counts. This enables a healthier lifestyle without giving into constant unhealthy cravings. Vegan recipes are very adaptable and tasty dishes can be prepared with half or less of the calorie and harmful fat counts.

- **Body Odor:**

  One of the important reasons that causes bad odor is the consumption of red meat. Since the vegan diet shuns the consumption of meat, the problem of bad odor does not arise.

- **Bad Breath:**

  In the same vein as body odor, the shunning of red meat and dairy also lessens bad breath. Bed breath and morning breath is significantly reduced through adopting a vegan diet.

- **Nails:**

  Abundance of nutrients in vegan diet leads to healthier and stronger nails. Nail health is often considered indicative of overall health and therefore is considered one of the most visible signs of health.

- **PMS:**

  The elimination of red meat and dairy from diet is considered to be effective in reducing the symptoms of PMS. The impact may be linked to a healthier system overall with reduced toxin buildup and resultantly lesser hormonal imbalances. However calcium intake should be taken care of and foods should be selected in a manner that does not encourage any deficiencies.

- **Allergies:**

Reduction of meat and dairy and eggs in the diet has been shown to have a positive impact on allergic symptoms. Simple allergies are often curbed by reduction of animal derived substances. Vegans report lesser congestions and runny noses. This may be due to the adequate provisions of vitamins and minerals in the diet that are helpful in boosting the immune system.

- **Hair care:**

Hair growth is promoted by the nutrient rich vegan diet. Following the vegan diet also helps in increasing the volume of the hair.

- **Migraines:**

Say no to constant migraines by adopting the vegan diet. Excessive sodium is often considered a culprit and at times dryness of the eyes can also contribute to migraines. Vitamin A and potassium rich diets can effectively keep such issues at bay.

- **Energy level:**

Since the vegan diet is rich in anti-oxidants, it helps in maintaining the energy levels of the body. The food is also fiber rich and aids in better metabolism thus keeping the energy levels high. Food that is easily digested does not contribute to bloating and constipation.

- **Longevity of life:**

Since following the vegan diet reduces the risks of many chronic diseases, it can be safely said that it promotes longevity of life. Research shows that vegans live for a longer time when compared with other vegetarians and non-vegetarians.

- **Cardiovascular Disease:**
Cardiovascular health is greatly improved through the elimination of red meats and full fat dairy from the diet. Red meats are higher in LDL cholesterol (low density lipoprotein) and when oxidized can lead to plaque growth of cholesterol in the arteries and veins resulting in blocked arteries and veins. These can heighten the risk of heart attacks and strokes. Various sources of protein in the vegan diet do not have high cholesterol levels and are easily digested. The various vitamins, phytochemicals and anti-oxidants present in vegan diet also help reduce the amount of bad cholesterol in the body.

- **Blood Pressure:**

  Blood Pressure maintenance is crucial to a healthy lifestyle. Magnesium is important for maintenance of blood pressure that is found abundantly in vegan diets. Vegan food is better for digestion and provides sustained sugar release through having lesser processed food. It also aids in balancing the levels of sodium in the body through provision of potassium in various foods. This balanced release of sugars keeps the blood glucose levels steady and effective removal of toxins from the body helps in maintaining healthy blood pressure and keeps related diseases at bay. Diet rich in whole grains can help effectively manage high blood pressure.

- **Type-2 Diabetes:**

  The vegan diet is more effective and easier to follow than the current recommendations doctors have for type-2 diabetes. The vegan diet has been known to be effective in reduction of likelihood of development of type-2 diabetes. Meaty and fatty diets are the prime culprits in the development of the body's resistance to the actions of insulin. Vegan or plant based diet is low fat, particularly in the minimal amounts of saturated fat that it contains. Due to the variety present in vegan diet, choices can be made in the selection of the healthiest foodstuff. This aids in keeping diabetes in check while at the same time not cutting essential nutrient requirements from diet. Vegan diet does not require measuring and weighing out of portions thus giving diabetic patients the ease of being able to eat to their fill without incurring any harm.

- **Prostate Cancer:**

  Vegan diet in lieu of the health benefits that it provides has been known to have positive impacts on the progression of diseases like prostate cancer. A study conducted showed that switching to vegan diet had a significant impact in regression of the disease. A study has shown that men who have switched to vegan diet in the earliest stages of cancer have shown significant reversal of the cancer. Vegan diet can thus also be helpful in the prevention of prostate cancer and allows for a very healthy life.

- **Breast Cancer:**

  Countries in which vegan diet is the norm and women are inclined to consume lesser meat and other animal products have shown to have a lower rate of breast cancer in comparison to those where more meat is consumed. Vegan women have 34% lower rates of breast, cervical and ovarian cancer. The cancer promoting growth hormone

IGF-1 is significantly higher in meat eaters as compared to vegans. The vegan diet helps in significantly reducing the level of IGF-1 in the blood stream thus hindering the progress of the disease. Vegan diet has been known to be effective in changing the behavior of around 500 genes, thus giving the body a better chance at fighting and preventing cancer. This is enabled through the dietary coercion given to the genes, activating those that are helpful in fighting and preventing cancer while deactivating those, which might be aiding in the development of the cancer.

- **Colon Cancer:**

  Switching to a diet filled with whole grains, fresh fruits and vegetables can also prevent Colon cancer. Since a vegan diet contributes significantly in reduction of risks from obesity, hypertension and diabetes, it helps in maintaining health. The coercive and proactive impacts that vegan diets have on genetics also help in enabling better preventive measures from cancer. Vegan diets are also rich in fibers (both soluble and insoluble) and help immensely in retaining digestive and bowel health. A healthy system keeps toxins at bay, and this in collusion with the genetic impact vegan diet has can greatly reduce the chances of developing colon cancer.

- **Arthritis:**

  Arthritis is the inflammation of joints and is a very painful affliction. The individuals suffering from arthritis have been known to find significant relief through elimination of dairy from their diet. A new research has indicated that a gluten-free diet combined with a vegan diet can be very effective in managing the condition of rheumatoid arthritis.

It is evident that the vegan diet is the one stop solution for many of your health issues. It promotes general well being as well as being an easy way of defending the body against various issues that can arise with a bad diet. Vegan diets have a whole host of nutritional value and are thus a very good life choice.

Brian Adams

Chapter 4: Nutritional Benefits of a Vegan Diet

A number of nutritional benefits can be achieved through developing of a well-balanced vegan diet. It is crucial that vegans should follow a diet filled with a wide variety of foods in order to achieve the full nutritional benefits. A selection of health benefits is stated below.

Carbohydrates

Carbohydrates are essential in order for provision of energy to the human body. Carbohydrates are broken down into glucose and crucial for a healthy diet. Without an adequate serving of carbohydrates in daily diet the body starts burning muscle tissue. Vegan diet includes a variety of food sources that are carbohydrate rich, which includes corn, bananas, whole grain cereals, white potatoes, sourdough bread and green peas.

Reduced Saturated Fats

Most meat and dairy rich diets include a high quantity of saturated fats that are considered the main culprits of various diseases. A vegan diet is low in saturated fats and therefore is extremely healthy. Vegan diets are excellent choices for individuals worried about cardiovascular health.

Protein

Protein is essential to good health and is one of the main building blocks of muscle, cartilage, blood, nails, hair and skin. Meat and dairy are considered the main sources of protein, but as a vegan diet completely cuts these sources out, it is crucial that these are replaced adequately. Vegan diet has many sources of protein that are adequate for a healthy and balanced diet. These sources include beans, nuts, lentils, and soy products.

Fiber

A high fiber diet is considered best for maintaining healthy bowels and maintenance of weight and blood sugar levels. Both soluble and insoluble fibers are present in abundance in vegan diet. Soluble fiber helps in lowering blood cholesterol and the maintaining of glucose levels. Insoluble fiber or roughage helps in maintaining a healthy digestive system and high fiber diets help in prevention of colon cancer. Insoluble finer can be found in whole wheat flour, wheat bran, beans, nuts and various vegetables like potatoes, cauliflower and green beans. Soluble fiber is present abundantly in oats, beans, barley, carrots, apples, and citrus fruits. Vegan diet contains a myriad of food products that contains both soluble and insoluble fiber and to maintain a healthy diet a wide variety of foods should be included.

Antioxidants

Antioxidants are crucial for maintenance of cell health and for the prevention of breakdown of cells. They help by destroying free radical that can damage healthy cells and consequently DNA. Cell damage can cause pre-mature aging and various health issues including a number of cancers and antioxidants are essential in preventing such damages. Vegan diet is extremely rich in antioxidant containing foods. Foods such as prunes, raspberries, strawberries, cranberries, blueberries, blackberries, walnuts, artichokes, pinto beans, kidney beans, and small red beans all include adequate amounts of antioxidants for a healthy diet. Antioxidants are directly related to the Vitamins ACE, all three are the best sources for antioxidants.

Phytochemicals

Phytochemicals are the broad reference terms used for the variety of compounds that are produced by plants. Phytochemicals are found in fruits, vegetables, grains, beans and a variety of other plants. A simple way to achieve adequate phytochemicals in daily nutrition is to eat through the colors, more commonly referred to as eating the rainbow. The phytochemical family contains antioxidants, flavonoids, flavones, isoflavones, phytonutrients, catechins, anthocyanidins, iso-thio-cyanates, carotenoids, allyl-sulphides, and polyphenols. Phytochemicals have a large role in maintaining health and thus are crucial inclusions in diet. They maintain immune systems, heart health, bones, muscles, skins, lung, and blood vessel health and are also considered helpful in prevention of formation of various cancers. Common phytochemicals include beta-carotene, lycopene, lutein, resveratrol, anthocyanidins, and isoflavones. In order to incorporate enough phytochemicals in diet, one can easily do so through color eating. Filling up on a variety of different vegetables and fruits can help in ingesting an adequate amount and variety of phytochemicals.

Magnesium

Magnesium is mineral that is crucial for the maintenance of various body functions. It aids in calcium absorption and therefore keeps bones strong, maintenance of blood pressure and thus keeping heart rhythm steady. Vegan diet is an excellent source of magnesium with nuts, seeds, beans, avocados, bananas, dried fruit, dark chocolate, and dark leafy greens being high in mineral content. In order to maintain healthy bones and overall well-being magnesium is a crucial component in healthy diet.

Magnesium deficiency is commonly indicated through a feeling of lethargy and adding the aforementioned foods in diet can help alleviate that.

Potassium

Potassium is a mineral that is responsible for balancing of water and acidity in the body and stimulates the kidneys for elimination of harmful toxins that are accumulated in the system. It also helps in regulation of blood pressure and thus protects the heart and reduces the risk of stroke through the ridding of excess sodium. It also reduces the risk for kidney stones and prevents bone loss. The normal requirements in a daily dose can be easily gained from a well-balanced diet. Vegan diet includes many ingredients that are excellent sources of potassium. Dark leafy greens, potatoes, squash, avocados, mushrooms, bananas, squash, white beans and lentils are all safe sources of potassium.

Vitamin A

Vitamin A is necessary for vision, boosting the immune system, skin health and gene transmission. Vitamin A is of crucial importance but it is essential that it should be ingested in a balanced way, as over-dosing can cause various health issues like jaundice, nausea, irritability, and vomiting and hair loss. Foods that are high in vitamin A are carrots, sweet potatoes, winter squash, lettuce, dried apricots, bell peppers, cantaloupe, mangoes and dark leafy greens. Vitamin A rich diet can prevent issues like night blindness and since it is antioxidant rich, gives the added benefits of damage prevention at a cellular level.

Vitamin C

Vitamin C is often considered to be amongst the most effective nutrients. It is considered to be responsible for protection against the various immune system deficiencies, prenatal health issues, cardiovascular diseases and various other benefits like skin health, eye health and prevention against stroke. Vitamin C is abundant in citrus fruits, green peppers, red peppers, strawberries, raspberries, blueberries, tomatoes, broccoli, white and sweet potatoes, dark leafy greens, mangoes, watermelons, winter squash, cantaloupes, Brussels sprouts, cabbages and cauliflowers. An adequate intake of vitamin C can boost the immune system effectively, keeping viruses like the common cold at bay.

Vitamin E

Vitamin E is a blanket term for eight naturally occurring nutrients and is very important for the maintenance of health. It is fat soluble and is an important source of antioxidants that prevents against free radical damage. It also helps in prevention of heart diseases through the prevention of oxidation of LDL cholesterol. Vitamin E also benefits skin, eyes, brain, and is also being considered to be helpful in the prevention of Alzheimer's disease. Vitamin E rich foods include dark leafy greens, grains, sunflower seeds, avocados and nuts like almonds and peanuts.

Vitamin K

Vitamin K is another class of naturally occurring nutrients and helps in blood clotting and prevention of excessive blood loss. It is not usually used in supplement form and thus a healthy diet can help maintain adequate levels of the nutrient. Vegan diet includes many sources like dark leafy vegetables including spinach, mustard greens, kale, beet greens, turnip greens, Swiss chard and broccoli.

Folate

Vitamin B complex is essential for a healthy system and is crucial to a well-balanced diet. This vitamin is often found in protein rich foods and by eliminating meat, vegan diet is often considered to be lacking in vitamin B and iron rich foods. This is however not the case; many foods in vegan diet are exceptionally rich in folates. These include red kidney beans, black eyed peas, dark leafy greens like turnip greens, Brussels sprouts, spinach and broccoli; various fruits and vegetables like avocados, papayas, cantaloupe, and oranges.

Vegan diet often provides a large number of nutrients and this is in lieu of its source ingredients, which are often not processed excessively. Natural sources of nutrients are always considered to be better than taking supplements. Medical health experts frown upon supplementing tablets for nutritious food. Most of the time people do not focus on eating balanced and healthy food and therefore end up relying on supplements to their diet. In the long run this is extremely harmful for the body as this can lead to toxic buildup of otherwise good nutrients and the body also loses its capacity for processing foods adequately. When food is nutritionally balanced the body functions well and health is shown to be markedly improved. The protein received from meat is considered complete, i.e. the amino acids in animal protein are complete. In contrast the plant proteins are often incomplete; therefore in order to have adequate intake of the amino acids combining proteins is considered to be effective. On the whole when vegans commit to the diet, they need to be conscious of the nutritional intake. By combining various sources of food vegans can eat better and do not develop any nutritional deficiencies that might occur due to cutting out dairy and meat.

Chapter 5: Tips to Get Started and Nutritional Health Concerns to Address

Before we jump into the recipes, we have some tips for those who are going to follow the Vegan diet for the first time. The pointers mentioned in this chapter should be borne in mind while following the vegan diet.

➤ Clean your refrigerator to get rid of meat, dairy products and egg products. Make sure to remove these ingredients from the pantry as well. This reduces the chances that you will get tempted to eat those products. Do not throw away the food items; donate them to the Salvation Army or to an orphanage. You will feel good about yourself, adding to the satisfaction of the deed!

➤ Shop smarter. By changing to a vegan diet, you incorporate many ingredients into your diet that keep very well. These include whole grains, dried fruits and nuts and thus buying them in bulk helps in saving money and keeping from frequent shopping trips for all your ingredients. Having dried fruits present in your pantry also keep you from snacking on unhealthy stuff. Visit organic farmers markets if possible and by going shopping around closing time can help you get some discounts on food. Even if you want to pick out fresh produce, an organic version is a far better option. Steer clear of tinned food where possible.

➤ Be wary while you switch over to meat substitutes like vegan meat and dairy substitutes like soy cheese, especially if you are choosing vegan diet to reduce your weight. Though these foods make the transition from a non-vegetarian to a vegan easier, they have a high fat and sodium content and help you gain few more pounds. Hence, always go for the organic version of these substitutes.

➤ Go at your own pace. It is essential that the switch from an omnivore to a completely vegan diet is made with conscious effort and in pace with the body's natural preference. A good way to wean off meat and dairy is to begin by singular substitution. One can start by substituting a single high consumption non-vegan product for a vegan substitute. Next one can crowd out unhealthy foods for healthier vegan substitutes and thus gradually reduce the amount of unhealthy foodstuff in the diet.

Substitution is easy in contrast with quitting cold turkey, as this allows the taste buds to settle and cravings to be managed.

➤ Evolve your diet on the basic idea of going vegan. The only rule that vegans really have to follow is the consumption of plant derived sources of food. It has no set rules on what you are supposed to eat and at what times. One can indulge their cravings through being experimental with vegan ingredients. Experimenting with a wide variety of foods can expand the palate. Since veganism stems from conscious consumption of resources and a satisfied palate makes the transition easier. Vegan diet also does not mean having bland food or a diet based solely on grains. A variety of vegan flavors can be combined to develop rich and fulfilling dishes that soothe both the palate and the conscience!

➤ Fretting on your daily intake of proteins will make you miserable and unable to commit to the lifestyle. It is as if you switch from counting calories to counting protein intake and this takes the fun out of eating. In order to keep this issue in check, make sure that major meals combine a variety of different whole grains, beans and nutrient rich vegetables like asparagus, cauliflower and broccoli. In addition to this you can also add vegan protein powder to milkshakes and smoothies.

➤ Make sure to incorporate a myriad of vegetables and fruits into regular diet. This helps in developing a nutrient rich daily diet that contains the essential vitamins, minerals, and antioxidants the body requires.

➤ Drink lots of water every day. Make sure you drink anywhere between six to twelve glasses of water in a day. Avoid drinking tap water as it may contain a lot of impurities. But, instead of opting for mineral or bottled water, invest in a good quality water purifier. This will be more monetarily feasible in the long run, and even leads to the less generation of waste as you avoid all the extra plastic from bottled water.

➤ Since the vegan diet eliminates the consumption of meat, one of the areas of concern is the reduction in the protein intake. Consumption of legumes and nuts ensures that the body gets the required amount of protein. Soy is another ingredient that is rich in protein. As a rule of thumb, every meal should have at least one legume, nut or soy product in it, in good quantities. Drizzling peanut oil on salad doesn't count as a good quantity, but topping a salad with a handful of nuts does!

➤ Beans are an integral component of the vegan diet. Do not opt for the canned version of beans, as they are loaded with high sodium content. If a recipe calls for canned beans, use regular beans, soaked in warm water overnight, drained and rinsed.

➤ While you are consuming fruits as a part of your diet, ensure that you do not consume melon along with the other fruits. Since melon gets digested before the other fruits and foodstuffs, it can result in heartburn and gas. If you want to add melon to your fruit salad, consume at least three fourths of the other fruit, before you start consuming the melon.

➤ Raw vegan foods are packed with all the essential nutrients and enzymes that the body needs. Include at least one green salad as a part of your meal. If you do not like the taste of raw vegetables, you can gently steam the salad or roast it a bit before consumption.

➤ Begin every day with a fruit. You could have a fruit salad, or some vegan pancake topped with some cut fruit or even vegan crepes with a side of fresh fruits. You can even add some fruit to your porridge.

➤ Consume fresh sprouts every day. Since they are packed with fiber, it helps in regulating the metabolism of the body and aids in the digestion of food.

- ➤ Choose the right kind of fat to cook your food. Try to avoid oils as much as you can, as they are nothing but empty calories. Avoid using refined oils to cook your food. Extra virgin olive oil can be a neutral substitute for these refined oils. Coconut oil is another healthy and viable substitute for refined oils.
- ➤ Say no to packaged and processed foods. Opt for whole and organic foods.
- ➤ Reduce your sugar intake by using substitutes like agave nectar or raw sugar. Avoid refined white sugar.
- ➤ Do not drink fruit juice. Fruit juices are a natural source of sugar and are devoid of the fiber that is present in the fruit. Hence, eat the fruits instead of consuming them in the juice form if you wish to derive the maximum benefits. If you really want to consume the juices, ensure that they are the "pulpy" version.
- ➤ Complement your diet with a suitable aerobic exercise. This will help you in losing those extra pounds soon. You can even start the day with some yoga poses or even perform a few sets of the sun salutation to ensure a healthy body and mind.

Health Concerns that need to be kept in mind with a Vegan Diet:

When thinking of adapting a vegan diet it is essential that a number of concerns should be addressed. Although plant based diets are quite nutrients dense, the concerns over such diets on being completely devoid of certain nutrients can become a cause for concern over the long run. Vegetables, fruits and whole grains and legumes contain within them a variety of vitamins and minerals. But at the same time certain nutrients although while being present in good quantity in vegan diets, tend to promote deficiencies. Some on the other hand are not so readily available in vegan diet. These include vitamin B12, calcium, iron, zinc and long chain fatty acids like EPA and DHA as well as the fat soluble vitamins A and D.

Availability of Vitamin B12

A deficiency of vitamin B12 can lead to a variety of health issues, as it is essential for the synthesis of DNA and red blood cells. It works to this goal together with Folate and a deficiency can lead to fatigue, anemia, neurological and psychiatric problems, lethargy, weakness, and memory loss. It can also lead to complications in pregnancy and potentially heighten the risk of heart disease. Vegan sources of B12 like seaweed, fermented soy and spirulina contain B12 analogs called cobamides and can essentially block the intake of B12, thus increasing the body's need of it. Amongst the only truly reliable vegan sources of B12 are foods that are fortified with the vitamin B12. These include plant milks, breakfast cereals and soy products. In order to ascertain that one is getting enough vitamin B12, consider taking a supplement. B12 supplement providing at least 10 micrograms B12 supplement providing at least 2000 micrograms should be taken. Try taking one a day if you are going for 10 microgram one and once weekly is enough for the 2000 one. Any supplement needs to be chewed or allowed to dissolve in the mouth to help increase absorption. Also, fortified foods containing at least three micrograms (mcg or µg) of B12, two or three times a day should be ingested. Over the years of experimentation with vegan diet, fortified foods and supplements have proven to be the best way to manage adequate intake of B12 and in maintaining optimal health. The recommended intake of vitamin B12 in the United States is 2.4 micrograms a day for ordinary adults and 2.8 micrograms for pregnant women and nursing mothers. In addition to this, increasing the levels of Folate is also recommended in order to reduce the levels of homocysteine that is linked to increased risks of heart disease. Therefore it is essential that intake of vitamin B12 through fortified foods and supplements be made a permanent part of vegan diet in order to avoid unnecessary risks.

Calcium Intake

A highly restricted diet as those of vegans places the level of calcium intake in jeopardy as the calcium bioavailability from plants is reduced due to their levels of oxalate and phytate. This is due to the fact that oxalate and phytate inhibit calcium absorption. However vegan diet has its benefits as the lower amount of animal proteins that they eat reduces the losses of calcium in the body. However if dietary calcium is too low, this results in inevitable loss from the bones; calcium being essential for various tasks such as blood clotting and important functions of the muscles and the nerves. It is recommended that in order to fulfill an adequate calcium intake such sources should be chosen that are high in calcium that is adequately absorbed. These include fortified soymilk with extra nutrients including calcium; tofu set with calcium, soy nut and soybeans. Vegetable sources include Chinese cabbage, bok-choy, broccoli, mustard greens, various collards, kale, and okra. In order to keep bone health and prevent too much loss of calcium from the bones, vegans should take care of including the essential sources listed above. Calcium is available in a variety of other vegetables as well but does not allow effective absorption die to the aforementioned high levels of oxalate (in the form of oxalic acid) and phytate. It is therefore crucial that foods that aid calcium absorption are chosen and relied upon for adequate calcium intake.

Iron Intake

Iron also faces the same issues in vegan diet as calcium. The bioavailability of iron in plants is lesser than that in animal protein. Absorption can be hindered due to other dietary staples for vegans like supplemental calcium. Non-heme iron is less readily absorbed than heme iron that is animal derived. Vegans often have lower store of iron than non-vegans but that does not mean that they have higher anemic rates. There are many vegan sources of iron which should be included in large quantities in diet, especially as most vegans prefer calcium fortified milk and tofu. Also avoiding coffee and tea an hour before, and two hours after meals can help increase the absorption of iron. This is due to the presence of tannins that inhibit the absorption of iron. Increase intake of iron through eating non-heme foods with foods containing vitamin C. This helps in increasing the absorption of iron. A number of legumes, grains, nuts and vegetables contain adequate amounts of iron. In addition, some sources like tomato sauce, broccoli and leafy greens are not only rich in iron but also in vitamin C. Using a cast iron skillet for cooking can increase the amount of iron in the food, especially when iron rich foods are cooked with vitamin C. Also do not rely on spinach as a main source of iron; it contains a very high level of oxalates that inhibit iron absorption. Thus through proper understanding of how non-heme Iron works, you can keep up the levels necessary for excellent health.

Zinc Availability

Zinc is often found as phytate in vegan ingredients and can thus inhibit absorption. The absorption of zinc is known to have decreased from 8% to 32% in vegans in comparison to omnivores. Zinc is a crucial mineral and is required by the body for over 50 different enzymes. Vegans do not suffer from outright zinc deficiency and it often happens that vegans actually have a greater intake of zinc than omnivores. This may partially be due to the concerns regarding the incurrence of deficiencies and in part due to having a varied diet, where a number of zinc rich foods are being used in daily diet. A number of cereals are fortified with zinc and also have no inhibitors thus being a very good source. Nuts, seeds and their butters, grains, leafy greens and beans all contain nice quantities of zinc. Zinc absorption can be increased through a variety of cooking methods. These include toasting nuts and seeds before using them, using fermented foods like sourdough bread and tempeh as well as foods leavened with yeast. Soak the grains before cooking and try to consume sprouted legumes and seeds. By following these simple ways, any concerns of zinc deficiency can be readily dismissed.

Bio-availability of Fatty acids (Omega-3 and Omega-6)

Plant foods do not contain within them sufficiently high amounts of omega 3 and omega 6, the fatty acids. Linoleic acid or omega 6 and alpha-linoleic acid (omega 3) are both considered essential, as the body cannot synthesize them and thus need to be obtained through diet. Long chain omega 3 fatty acids like EPA (Eicosapentaenoic acid) and DHA (Docosahexaenoic acid) play a protective and therapeutic role in a wide range of diseases such as cancer, asthma, cardiovascular disease, ADHD, depression, and autoimmune diseases, such as rheumatoid arthritis. Some EPA is converted into other molecules that can help in the reduction of inflammation, blood clotting, blood pressure, and cholesterol. EPA's are found in very small quantities in seaweed. DHA's are the major components of the grey matter in the brain and is also part of the retina and cell membranes. Alpha-linoleic acid is a short chain fatty acid and is found in larger quantities in soy, walnuts, camelina oil, canola oil, and in flax, hemp, and chia seeds and their oils. In light of it being and essential fatty acid, it is crucial that foods high in alpha-linoleic acid be consumed daily. The body can effectively convert alpha-linoleic acid into EPA and EPA into DHA. Alpha-linoleic acid is quite effective in its conversion to EPA but the body requires large amounts of Alpha-linoleic acid to produce the necessary amounts of DHA. It is recommended that in order to minimize the risks associated with deficiencies, vegans should consider using a DHA supplement. One should be careful of ALA; the omega-6 fatty acid can induce eye damage and therefore food oils like soy, sunflower, corn, sesame, safflower and most vegetable oil blends should be used in cooking too often. These are high in omega 6 and oils like peanut, canola, avocado, and olive are low in omega 6 and should be used instead. Vegans on an average meet 50-60% of the recommended ALA dietary requirements without meal planning. In order to increase the intake, around 0.5 grams of raw ALA should be added to the daily diet. This amounts to an average of 6 grams English walnuts (3 halves) 1/4 teaspoon of flaxseed oil, ½ table spoon canola oil, or 1 teaspoon ground flaxseeds. Foods with a higher level of omega 3 acid should be preferred. In the case of flaxseeds the omega 6 to the omega 3 ratio is 1:4. They are the most concentrated source of alpha-linoleic acid and should be used in ground form or as oil. One tablespoon of ground flaxseeds contains 1.6 grams of Alpha-linoleic acid and one teaspoon of flaxseed oil contains 2.5 grams of Alpha-linoleic acid. You can also use chia seed oil as it is also a good source of Alpha-linoleic acid. Dried chia seeds have 5 g of ALA per ounce, with an omega-6 to omega-3 ratio of 1:3.

Absorption and Synthesis of Vitamin A

Vitamin A can easily be included in the diet due to its high content presence in a variety of fruits and vegetables. The trick is to choose orange vegetables and fruits that are high in vitamin A. However a lacking of the vitamin can develop, as the daily intake of recommended amounts is necessary for the actual effective availability of the vitamin. The issue with taking in a number of vegetables and fruits is the high consumption of oxalates that can in turn reduce the absorption of a number of nutrients and can increase the risk of developing deficiencies. Since Vitamin A is fat soluble and it requires to be utilized in a manner that increase the absorption on a daily basis. One of the best options to increase the amount of vitamin A intake is to utilize juices from orange fruits and vegetables. Since plants contain beta-carotene, in order for conversion into vitamin A to be effective, the human body needs a greater amount. High oxalate greens in blended form with other vitamin rich vegetables can cause issues over a long run if used too frequently. High oxalate foods like spinach, Swiss chard and beet greens can lead to kidney stones if used on a regular basis in raw blended form. Since they act as inhibitors, it is crucial that if one is worried about any deficiencies in terms of intake and absorption of necessary minerals and vitamins to understand how various vegetables work in light of their composition. A long-term deficiency in vitamin A can cause night blindness or Nyctalopia, but this is rare in developed nations and even more in vegans. Lower absorption of vitamin A can occur but if a diet is well-balanced and well planned, any inhibitor in absorptions can easily be overlooked due to the more than adequate amounts being introduced in the daily diets of vegans.

Absorption and Synthesis of Vitamin D

Vitamin D is often known as the sun vitamin and it is so because of the human body's capacity to synthesize the vitamin through exposure to the sun. It is in fact a vitamin that is quite rare in food. It is only found in certain fatty fish and apart from people that eat fatty fish on a daily basis, vitamin D deficiency can be seen without exception in omnivores, vegetarians and vegans. Vitamin D is quite crucial in various functions of the body and maintenance of good health. It aids the absorption of calcium in the bones thus keeping issues like osteoporosis at bay. The deficiency of vitamin D can lead to increased risk for cancer, muscle weakness, multiple sclerosis and depression. One of the best perks of living in this age is the availability of a number of fortified foods that are suitable for vegans and omnivores alike. Since the availability of vitamin D is subject upon so many clauses, reliance solely on the sun can be harmful in the long run. The absorption and synthesis decrease with age and anything that blocks UV rays like sunscreen and clouds can hamper with vitamin synthesis. For vegan the best options are to try fortified cereals and fortified vegan milks like those made from soy, almonds, hempseed and rice.

Vegan diet can be a very healthy option, but it is essential like any other diet plan that one follows certain guidelines that keep the endeavor healthy and completely devoid of any unnecessary health risks. Vegans need to keep in mind the overall nutritional benefits of adopting the diet in light of the diversity of the diet. This means that the diet needs to include a very large variety of ingredients from all the food groups. By making sure that multiple foods from every group are being included on a regular basis, you can make sure that you do not suffer from any nutritional pitfalls. Include a number of fortified ingredients in your daily diet. This can include fortified cereals, breads, milks (including almond and soy milk) and soy derived products such as tofu. Choose low fat sources of protein, as these are healthier options especially while aiming for weight loss. Do not over compensate for the loss of one nutrient source by substituting the near alternative in excess. Substitution from non-vegan to vegan should be done in accordance with bioavailability of the nutrients. Take into account the nutritional content and the effectiveness of absorption of the products. Checking the nutritional values of any packaged foods that you consume is a great way to ascertain the amount of nutrition you would gain. If you feel like you are lacking in certain nutrients such as vitamin D or vitamin B12, consider taking a supplement. Women during pregnancy and lactation should follow a dietitian's advice. Teenagers and young children should also follow diets recommended by good dietitians in order to keep nutritional deficiencies at bay. This holds true for any age if the diet that you choose is restrictive. In the case that you follow a vegan diet for losing weight, be sure of the nutritional benefits in correlation to the amount/serving sizes that you choose. Also, vegan diet is naturally low in fat and thus allows you to lose more weight. Therefore do not limit yourself to far too strict a diet, this will only serve to disrupt your natural metabolism and make you more prone to hunger pangs and giving into unhealthy indulgences.

Vegan Diet and Weight Loss

The perks of using vegan diet as a choice for weight loss is the amazing diversity that it holds within its humble name. Common misconceptions term it as rabbit food and nutritionally lacking, but the truth could not be farther. In fact many of the essentials while considering weight loss are often available only in plant sourced diets. A common issue with weight loss is that once you have changed your diet to drop the pounds, it stays that way only until that specific diet is followed. Once you go back to your regular diet, even with a controlled eating and portioning does not help you keep the pounds down. The easier and healthier way to not only shed the weight but to also increase your chances of keeping weight gain at bay is to choose your diet as a lifestyle choice. A vegan diet is amongst the best options if fluctuating weight gain has been a problem for you. Everyone knows the struggle of giving into indulgences and cravings and here is where we weak humans fail spectacularly! In order to make sure that you are on the right path, the best advice that you can receive is to find balance. Push yourself towards the right direction but do not over stress yourself. A vegan diet is amazing in the light that it can actually help you indulge in amazing dishes with a significantly less degree of calories to worry about.

Another added benefit of choosing the vegan diet is the overall benefits that can be gained through focusing on what you put in your body. A vegan diet can also help stave off the overindulgence that modern day life is prone to in the garb of ease. Sodium loaded foods, prepackaged and from take outs adds to the list of unhealthy and over used oils, excessive usage of meat in every meal and in the long run having absolutely no balance that an omnivore diet actually speaks of.

The vegan diet lays its emphasis on the balance of lifestyle choices. Once a vegan diet is adopted, following the basics of a healthy lifestyle tend to become second nature. This is due to the fact that vegan diet in lieu of its structure enables an individual to be extremely aware of every meal plan. Vegans often opt to eat a combination of foods in every single meal. By combining the basic four food groups of veganism (fruits, vegetables, grains and legumes), better health benefits can be achieved. This happens due to the overall interaction vegan foods have with each other. It aids everywhere, from helping in easy digestion to enabling the body to synthesize necessary nutrients from the forms present in vegan ingredients. Many issues that contribute to weight gain include the overall physical acceptance the body has for various foods, the overall eating habits and resultant nutritional value and the portioning of foods. Various foods can cause allergies and lower tolerance to certain foodstuffs can simply eliminate a number of otherwise necessary (nutrient wise) ingredients from the diet. Vegan foods provide a large variety of alternative sources and can thus better accommodate for any nutritional pitfalls one might encounter. By eating a number of healthy nutritionally diverse sources for all three meals, a vegan diet provides a better overall intake of necessary nutrients.

In light of wanting to lose weight with a vegan diet, one needs to be sure that a blind following of the suggested intake is actually an obstruction to the end goal. Vegan food pyramids are often constructed with the basic requirements in mind. Often the suggested servings are developed in light of individuals requiring optimal nutritional gain and at time increasing their weight (muscle mass, internal strength, bone density etc.). Weight loss can be achieved through the development of one's own variation of the vegan food pyramid. Opting for lower numbers of servings is one way to go. By staying in the lower range of suggested servings, weight loss can be achieved without incurring any nutritional deficiencies. It is an issue of *'prime importance'* that you do not simply substitute your diet. This point has been reiterated many times and for the simple reason that soy meats and cheeses are often high in fat and sodium, which is less than ideal if it is a weight loss that is an end goal.

The best ways to actually jump start your digestion and metabolism is through experimenting with whole grains. The complex carbohydrates that are provided by whole grains (try and buy dried, organic and whole grains) are amazing for the energy levels and also keep those nasty hunger pangs at bay. In order to find the whole grains that work for you best try and experiment with a number of them. Whichever one suits you and your digestion better is the one that you can use more frequently. Natural whole grains move through the digestive track slowly in comparison to pseudo cereals. In order to be able to lose weight, one needs to feel fuller for longer.

Steer clear of juices; fruits in their *actual* form are amazing sources of vitamins, fiber and are water rich. You do not need to drink them for maximum impact. Store bought fruit juices also contain an obscenely high amount of simple sugars in order to make them taste palatable. They are also often made from concentrates and are thus detrimental to your weight loss goals. Drink lots of water and cut out fizzy drinks completely. As mentioned before, even juices do not work towards your goal especially if they are store bought. Instead try some homemade smoothies, that are far healthier and help you pack in a lot of nutrients in one serving.

Include nuts and seeds into your diet as they provide a number of healthy fats that are extremely important for your health. Include both raw and toasted nuts for enzymes and increased protein.

When you aim to start your vegan diet, it is best that a few simple guidelines are followed. These help in transitioning from your existing dietary lifestyle easier.

Choose the right day to start your diet. It should not be around a time when festivities, parties and celebrations are planned.

If you are obligated to go to dinners and parties and eat outside, make sure that you choose the healthier options. A lot of restaurants now serve completely vegan options. There is no reason to become a hermit just because you are changing your diet!

While travelling, look through the local cuisine and choose the vegan options that would suit you best. Also choose non-dairy vegetarian options while flying.

Initially try to plan the diet for a short time in order to help transitioning. The body's metabolism can get used to the diet pattern and help you lose weight in about 3 weeks.

Developing a comprehensive chart of meals for the 3 weeks should help getting on track with the nutritional requirements. By charting meals for a short time you can enable the body to accept the dietary change and can allow for a basic guideline to exist throughout your diet regimen.

Weigh and measure yourself before you start the diet. Keep track of both your weight and measurements as you progress. This is crucial as weighing alone can be unhelpful. It has often been seen that progressing on a well-balanced diet often helps build muscle mass that is extremely helpful in reducing bad fat and toning the body. But muscle is denser than fat and the scale might say so. By keeping track of concurrent measurements you can notice the changes in the body better.

Maintaining a journal of foods that you've eaten during the day and also your weekly progress can help in sustaining your regimens. Progress can make anyone feel good and it is essential that you realize your progress. Also make note of the overall energy that you have and any feel good factors that you would associate with your diet change.

Be wary of the portion sizes. It often happens that a switch to the vegetarian meal plans leads people to believe they need to gorge on every meal. This only ends up adding extra calories to your intake. Vegetarian food pyramids are often built for weight gain, so if you are following one stay at the lower spectrum of serving sizes and numbers per day. Keeping yourself from overeating is crucial. The best way to do that is through making sure that you are partaking of a variety of foods every day. This helps in giving you essential nutrients and complex carbohydrates which will fill you up for longer, making it impossible to overeat.

To get over cravings, stock up your home and office with healthy snacks such as crackers, puffed rice, peanuts, almonds, other dry fruits, and smoothies. Try for natural and raw ingredients where possible and reduce your intake of simple sugars. This helps keep the hunger pangs at bay.

Brian Adams

Chapter 6: Foods to Eat, Foods to Avoid & Replacements for Common Non- Vegan Foods

Foods vegans can eat

- All fruits: Citrus fruits like oranges, sweet limes, lemons; all kinds of berries, like strawberries, blue berries, black berries; all melons like, water melon, musk melon; and other fruits like, bananas, mangos, apples, cherries, etc.

- All veggies: All green veggies like, spinach, Swiss chard, kale, broccoli, lettuce, cabbage; root vegetables like, potatoes, sweet potatoes, carrots, radishes; and other vegetables like cauliflower, onions, tomatoes, mushrooms, garlic, etc.

- All grains: All grains can be consumed as long as they are not too refined, like, wheat, rice, oats, quinoa, corn, barley, faro, teff, millet, sorghum, rye, etc.

- All legumes: Legumes are the main source of protein for vegans and are very important in a vegan's diet. Each meal should contain a legume like, soybeans, chickpeas, kidney beans, fava beans, black beans, white beans, black eyed peas, pinto beans, etc.

- All seeds: Along with legumes, seeds are also one of the important sources of proteins and should be consumed in good quantities. We consume seeds like sesame seeds, coriander seeds, flax seeds, mustard seeds, poppy seeds, etc.

- All nuts: Belonging to the protein rich food category, nuts are very important too. Nuts are extremely easy to include in the diet as you can roast and drop a bunch in salads or eat them as it is, without the need to cook them! Some of the most popular and healthy nuts you can consume are, peanuts, cashew nuts, walnuts, almonds, chestnuts, Brazilian nuts, macadamia nuts, candlenuts, pine nuts, pistachios, hazelnuts, etc.

- Canned Foods: All the aforementioned food items can be consumed in their natural form. Canned and items can be consumed, but as mentioned earlier, it is better if you avoid those.

- Whole Wheat Breads: Traditionally, most whole wheat breads are made without eggs and milk, unless they are specifically milk breads or egg breads, so it is safe to consume most bakery made breads.

- Pastas: Most of the store bought pasta is vegan, unless you opt for fresh pasta. Fresh pasta usually contains eggs and should be avoided.

- Meat and Dairy Substitutes. Certain dairy substitutes are excellent for inclusion in the diet. These include soymilks, tofu, almond milk and almond butters. You can consume meat substitutes made from soy but since they are high in sodium, use them quite sparingly. If you are attempting to go vegan, you need to re-teach your palate instead of relying on substitutes.

Foods Vegans Can Not Eat

- All Animal Meats: This list includes all kinds of meats like, bacon, pork, ribs, steaks, veal, lamb, etc.; all poultry like, chicken, pheasant, duck, turkey, fowl, etc.; all fishes like, snapper, mackerel, tuna, salmon, sea bass, trout; and all sea food like, prawns, shrimp, lobsters, crabs, calamari, oysters, squid, octopus, etc.

- **The basic principal that vegans follow is that "if it moves, you don't eat it!"**

- All kinds of dairy and dairy products: Vegans do not consume any kind of milk that has been derived from any animal like cow, goat, camel, buffalo or yak. Also, vegans do not consume any product made from the milk of animals like, cheese, yogurt, cream, ice cream, etc.

- All animal eggs: Vegans do not consume any eggs got from animals, like chicken eggs, fish eggs or duck eggs or products derived from eggs, like mayonnaise, egg noodles, pasta, hollandaise sauce, certain canned soups, salad dressings, certain lollipops, marshmallows, marzipan, etc.

- Honey: Though a lot of vegans do consume honey, most of the stricter vegans stay off honey as it is derived from bees.

- All animal by-products: This can be a very long list of items, and most vegans strive to avoid the items on this list.

o *Animal based broths*: A lot of animal based broths like a chicken broth or a beef broth is used as a base for a lot of soups, including a lot of pre-made "vegetarian" soups.

o *Gelatin:* Made from the skins, tendons, sinews and hooves of horses and cows, gelatin is used in a lot of desserts like soufflés and mousses and a lot of store bought candy and other products like marshmallows, Jell-O, gummy bears etc. It is also advisable to avoid prepackaged salted peanuts, as a lot of manufacturers add some gelatin to the peanuts as an additive.

  ▪ If you want to make vegan versions of these products or any products that contain gelatin, just substitute gelatin for equal amounts of agar-agar and you will be good to go!

o *Lac Bug*: Resin extracted from the lac bug is what gives most of the store bought candy a shiny outer glaze. This glaze, commonly referred to as confectioner's glaze, is actually a resin extracted from a lac bug. So, avoid all store bought candy!

o *Whey (or Whey Powder):* Derived from milk, whey is often used to make certain whey products like ricotta cheese and whey butter and is also used as an additive in many breads, pastries and crackers.

o *Casein:* Casein is also derived from milk and is used in the cheese making process, in protein supplements and in a lot of dental processes. Some of the soy cheeses also contain some quantities of casein in them, so read the labels before you purchase soy cheese!

o *White Sugar:* Before you protest saying sugar is derived from plants, read on! A lot of sugar refineries use bone char from animals to give the sugar a bright white color. So, even though sugar is not an animal product, it indirectly ends up being one.

o *Omega 3 Fatty Acids:* Some of the fruit juices, like orange juice, are fortified with some extra omega 3 fatty acids, which are derived from fish! So, make it a point to read all the labels and ingredient lists carefully before purchasing any product.

Substitutes for Common Foods

- Vegan Substitutes for Meat: You can use products like vegan burgers, vegan ribs, vegan sausages, Tofurkey roast, vegan chicken breasts, etc., to substitute for meaty items in your diet. These products make the transition from non-vegetarian to vegan easy, as these products offer your taste buds a level of familiarity, making it easy for you to adjust. The consumption of these products also ensures that there is no lapse in your resolve and you do not fall back to eating meat. If you do not like to consume these hybrid products, there are a variety of vegetables that make an excellent substitute for most meats. Some of the vegetables are:

  o *Tofu*: Technically not a vegetable, but it makes for a delicious substitute for some of the lighter meats like, chicken, crab and fish.

  o *Mushroom:* If you want to have the delicious and earthy flavors of lamb, try consuming some umami mushrooms. They are healthy and satiating without the drawbacks of meat.

- o *Eggplant:* With a rich meaty taste, eggplant is one of the first vegetables that any new vegan consumes to make the transition easy!

- o *Potatoes:* Potatoes are extremely satiating and make an ideal replacement for some good old meat. A lot of people write them off as a side dish, but in reality, potatoes make for an amazingly delicious and healthy main dish!

- Vegan dairy substitutes: One of the biggest sacrifices that people think they are making while following the vegan diet is giving up dairy products. After all, most desserts have large quantities of dairy in them, and who wants to give up dessert? Well, dairy substitutes, like almond milk, soymilk, hemp milk, soy cheese, tofu, soy yogurt, soy cheese, etc., will help make your life easier. You can make delicious desserts with these substitutes, without compromising on taste, like vegan coconut ice cream, soy ice cream, chocolate almond milk pudding, etc.

  - o If a recipe calls for one cup buttermilk, substitute it by combining one cup soymilk and one tablespoon of distilled white vinegar, and use as you would use the buttermilk.

- o To substitute whipped cream, there are various non-dairy whipping topping available in all specialty baking stores and kosher stores.

- Vegan egg substitutes: If a recipe calls for an egg, you can substitute it by mixing 2 tablespoons of hot water with 1 tablespoons of flax seed meal. Combine the flax seed meal and hot water in a small bowl and leave to soak for about 5 minutes or so, stirring every few minutes. Then, use the mixture in place of the egg.

- To prepare scrambled egg: If you crave some good scrambled egg, this is no reason for you to cheat on your diet! Just follow this simple hack to make a delicious scrambled egg substitute in no time:

  - o Take some tofu and break the tofu into smaller pieces using and egg scrambler.

  - o Heat some olive oil in a pan and lightly fry the tofu in it. Once the tofu has browned a little, add some chopped red peppers, chopped green onions, some salsa and some salt to taste.

Brian Adams

Chapter 7: Sample Vegan Diet Plans and Exercises for Beginners

To begin with, aspiring vegans should not be daunted by the prospect of replacing regular meals with vegan options. One of the easiest ways to do so is to reinvent commonly eaten recipes with vegan ingredients and prioritize the vegan meals that you have already been enjoying. This can be done with three simple steps.

Incorporate a greater number of proteins and vegetables in the vegan meals that you already eat and enjoy taste wise. This can act as a baseline for the foods you may like to eat and give you a baseline for the kind of food shopping that you need to do.

Think of three meals that you make on a regular basis and consider being a staple of your diet. Break down the ingredient list and separate the non-vegan ingredients. Substitute these with your choice of tofu, beans and/or vegetables of your choice. Use soy milk products in place of dairy and develop new vegetarian recipes out of the ones that you already love and cook often.

Next you can go through some vegetarian recipes that you might want to try out. You could try some exotic curries and dishes that feature vegetables as staple ingredients. Experiment with various dishes and tweak them in accordance with your taste preferences. Just make sure to add a variety of completing vegetables and grains to the mix in order to make them wholesome and nutritious.

By creating a meal plan on your taste preferences, it is easier to transition from non-vegan diet to completely vegan. You can ease off the meat and dairy and transition to vegetarian before achieving the end goal of veganism. Begin with easy substitution and vegan meals that you already prefer.

It is crucial that when following a vegan diet, one should have an adequate intake of the four major food groups that form the vegan eat-well plate. These four food groups consist of fruits, legumes, whole grains and vegetables.

The recommended fruit servings are 3 or more a day. The estimated ideal serving size consists of 1 medium piece of fruit, ½ a cup of cooked fruit and 4 ounces of juice. Fruits are crucial to the daily diet as they are rich in fiber, beta-carotenes and vitamin

C. Include at least one serving of citrus fruits in daily recommended eating.

The recommended serving of legumes is 2 or more a day. A standard serving of legumes includes ½ cup cooked beans, 4 ounces of tofu or tempeh, and 8 ounces of soymilk. Legumes include beans, peas and lentils and products derived from these basic foods. These include soy products like soymilk, tempeh and tofu. Since lentils are high in protein, iron, calcium and vitamin B they need to be included in daily diet and major dishes can be constructed with them as central ingredients.

Whole grains should be included in diet with 5 or more servings a day. One serving amounts to ½ cup of hot/cooked cereal or cooked rice, 1 ounce dry cereal and 1 slice of bread. Whole grains include whole wheat, rice, pasta cereal, corn and tortillas, millet, buckwheat, oats, barley, and bulgur. The choice for whole grains is quite varied and thus makes it easier to adapt them into a variety of recipes. Due to the high nutritional content of whole grains they are ideal as mains and a variety of exotic dishes feature fulfilling and tasty recipes.

The fourth food group consists of vegetables and it is suggested that an intake of 4 or more servings a day is necessary for good diet. A standard serving size includes 1 cup of raw vegetables and ½ cup of cooked vegetables. Vegetables in lieu of their color have different kinds of nutritional highlights. It is thus recommended that you eat the rainbow, including all the different kinds of vegetables in to your daily diet. Packed with vitamins, beta-carotenes, riboflavin, iron, calcium and fiber, vegetables constitute a very important part of vegan diet. Leafy greens also act as great fillers and make the meal more fulfilling.

Sample Menus:

For breakfast you can have 3 oatmeal and blueberry pancakes with maple syrup topping, orange juice preferentially calcium fortified, and fresh fruit. For lunch you could try whole wheat pita stuffed with sliced tomatoes, carrot sticks, lettuce, cucumbers and hummus. For dinner try a Chinese stir-fry over brown rice; add tofu chunks, broccoli, and sweet peas in pods, water chestnuts, and Chinese cabbage (bok choy) in the stir fry, have cantaloupe chunks drizzled with fresh lemon juice for dessert and for a snack try dried figs.

For breakfast try 1 cup oatmeal with cinnamon, shredded almonds and raisins, ½ cup fortified soymilk flavored if you want, 1 slice toast with 1 tablespoon almond butter, and ½ grapefruit. Lunch can consist of Bean burritos (black beans in corn tortillas, topped with chopped lettuce, tomatoes, and salsa, spinach salad with tahini-lemon dressing). For dinners go with 1 cup baked beans, 1 cup steamed collard greens drizzled with lemon juice, baked sweet potato and for dessert try baked apple. You could snack on Banana soymilk shake.

Breakfast can consist of a hot cereal of rolled oats, an apple and a handful of walnuts (whether in the cereal or on the side). For lunch try a hearty serving of lentil soup and 1 ½ cups of mixed greens salad. For dinner, go for a veggie burger with vegan cheese. Complement this with 2 cups of mixed greens salad combined with a cup of a variety of vegetables of your choice (include green peppers, cucumbers, onions etc.) For dessert try a roasted pear and non-dairy yoghurt. Snacks can be comprised of non-dairy fruit yoghurt.

Breakfast can comprise of tofu scramble with salsa, and orange juice. For lunch try a teriyaki wrap; combine celery, cucumber and carrot sticks and add to it a serving of beans of your preference. Add teriyaki sauce for taste and wrap in a whole wheat tortilla. You can add a small fruit salad as dessert. For dinner try a black bean enchiladas and a side of spinach topped with sesame seeds, vinegar and tamari. Prepare a smoothie with strawberries and non-dairy milk for dessert.

Try vegan toaster pops for breakfast with plain non-dairy yoghurt and a small pear. For lunch go for brown rice and a veggie bowl. This could be made with Indian curry recipes or you could go for Thai vegetable curry with coconut milk. For dinner try roasted vegetable tamale with a side of 2 servings of leafy greens salad. Have fresh fruits for dessert and snack on a handful of nuts of your choice.

For breakfast you could try cornmeal pancakes, orange juice and lemon poppy scone. Go for a pasta salad or choose a salad given in this book. Complement it with flavored soy yoghurt and some fresh fruit. For dinner you could try a delicious vegan hot and sour soup with toasted garlic whole wheat bread and fresh fruit as a dessert. For a snack you could go with crackers and a nice dip.

Make yourself some apple pancakes for breakfast and try a nice smoothie. For lunch you could try a bean burrito and a nice healthy helping of greens salad. For dinner try something exotic like vegan curry Kofte and Indian flatbread. Try a pear sorbet as a dessert and for a snack go for fresh fruits.

Blueberry pancakes for breakfast can be complemented with a lovely bowl of fresh fruits and honey. For lunch try a vegan burger and a large salad combining fresh vegetables and greens. Try a red lentil and butternut squash soup for dinner and choose a side dish of spicy sweet potato sticks. If you really want to indulge, try a vegan chocolate cake for dessert and snack on a handful of dried nuts.

For breakfast try some fortified cereals or muesli. Pair it with fresh fruits and a fresh squeezed juice. Try a couscous salad for lunch and try a side of a mix lentil kebab. For dinner try a corn chowder and whole wheat bread as a side. Dessert can comprise of a carrot cake with vegan ice cream. Skip the snacking if you are going to indulge in a heavy dessert.

Blueberry oatmeal waffles coupled with a soy or coconut milk smoothie for breakfast. Lunch can comprise of another salad variation with brown rice, heaped with leafy greens. For dinner go for sandwiches and a side of garlicky baked potatoes. Mojito Fresh Fruit salad for dessert can be a fresh choice and a break from a heavy dessert option.

From the above sample menus, you can see that there are almost infinite combinations that you can derive from the humble vegan origins. Even as you aim to lose weight you can indulge in a choice of desserts as the vegan varieties have a significantly lesser amount of calories than their non-vegan or dairy counterparts. Vegan diet includes a number of fresh ways you can use the ingredients and you can try any number of combinations. The combinations given above are but a simple outline for what you can try. Choose according to your own taste and preferences. Look through our chapters on various recipes and try out a few. Develop a combination that works best for you. Initially you can use a few tried and tested combinations that you prefer taste wise to wean yourself off meat. By developing a set meal plan for the initial weeks, you can be less temped to sneak anything non-vegan. The consistency of your diet does depend on how good your food tastes, so going the extra mile is always worth the effort. After all you are what you eat!

Exercises that you could try for weight loss:

Weight loss cannot solely be achieved through a vegan diet plan. You have to remember that you are still consuming a large number of calories and a variety of simple and complex sugars, proteins and other nutrients. The body therefore is not going to simply start shedding the excess fat. In order to focus the body on shedding unhealthy fat, vegan diet needs to be complemented with exercise. Once the body is forced into metabolizing the excess fat, you will start losing weight. A vegan diet is very effective in the manner that it does not have very high saturated fat contents and is quite low in sodium. If you cut down on fats and high content starch foods, you can jump start your weight loss by losing the excess or retained fluids. Vegan diet is more fulfilling and even when you might be eating a higher amount of calories than before, but adequate exercise and the unprocessed nature of the majority of vegan foods do not induce fat retention.

Once you start with weight loss regimens, make sure that you exercise enough to burn 500 calories more than you intake. This helps in starting your weight loss. Also be careful to pace yourself. If you don not exercise regularly then make sure to start gradually in order to not do yourself any harm.

Start with warming up and allow your body to ease into the regimen you set for yourself. Warm up for around 10 to 15 minutes before every work out. This will help you get your heart rate up. The warm up is a preamble of the workout that should work up a good sweat.

Choose exercises that keep your heart rate up for the better part of 30 minutes. Amongst the best exercises for weight loss are cardio and strength training. The best way to lose weight is to sweat for at least an hour past your warm up. This helps in losing the requisite calories and also aids in developing necessary muscle tone.

You can also try interval training. This is amongst the best ways to exercise for weight loss, as it provides necessary bursts of energetic workout without tiring you. The necessary push is achieved through the high energy work out bursts. This enables a greater burnout of calories.

Cardio:

Cardio exercise can include running, jumping rope, plyometric and stair-master.

Running:

You can choose to do this exercise outdoors or indoors as this is one of the easiest and most reliable choices when it comes to exercising for weight loss. Start with a pace and time spend that you are comfortable with. You could choose the treadmill or go outside. Try and run outside in the better weather, as this will give you the added benefit of soaking up some sun that enables vitamin D synthesis. Running is also good for your overall wellbeing as it provides much needed relaxation from the stress of a busy lifestyle. A good warm up gives your body extra needed stamina and you can slowly build your time and speed. If you choose running than be sure to be regular with it; try combining sprints and jogs as they act as great fat burners. Interval training on the treadmill an also act as a good fat burner. Try 15 second sprints followed by 40 seconds rest.

Jumping Rope:

Jumping rope makes for an excellent accompaniment as well as an amazing individual workout. This exercise is amongst the best for individuals who are stressed for time and need to fit in greater effectiveness into a smaller time scale. Try going in accordance with your own pace. Whatever intensity works for you should be the one that you start with. Slowly build up your stamina for jumping rope and add to the overall time frame that you would do this exercise. Also you can do interval training with jump rope. Try about 30 to 80 jumps with one minute rest. You could also try about 50 jumps in between any other cardio or strength training that you might be doing.

Jumping Jacks or Plyometric:

We are suggesting that you do the jumping jack exercise as this is one of the best exercises to get your heart rate elevated as well building up stamina for any more challenging exercises that you may choose to do in the future. Jumping jacks can be done in intervals and are excellent as filler in workouts. For novices this exercise is amongst the best as it requires no extra equipment. You have to begin with stretches as a warm up exercise in order to avoid any injury. Assume a straight position, with your arms at your side and feet together. Bend your knees a few degrees and jump a few inches into the air. When you are in the air, take your legs out to the sides about 15 inches width or slightly wider. When you are moving your legs outwards, elevate your arms up over your head; makes sure that the arms are slightly bent throughout the in-air movement. Land with your feet shoulder width or wider and with arms slightly bent simultaneously have your hands meet above your head. Repeat the process for anywhere from 30 to 100 repetitions.

Stairmaster:

For the Stairmaster, you would need some equipment and it is best done in the gym. This is however amongst the best fat burners and should be done around two to three times a week with a session lasting around 30 minutes. You can try both the high intensity interval training and the low intensity steady-state cardio. Both are amazing for fat burning and as is the case with any other exercise; start with a workout that you can manage and gradually increase the intensity. The Stairmaster is very good for glutes and thighs and incorporate in some glute kickbacks to target your rear.

Strength Training Exercises:

Squats and Overhead Weight Presses:

Start by standing with your feet shoulder-width apart. Hold a 5-pound weight in each hand at shoulder height with your elbows bent. Palms should be facing forward. Lower yourself into a squat (make sure your knees do not go past the toes); hold this position for around 45 seconds. Focus the weight through heels to stand up, pumping the weights overhead. Return to the starting position. Do 4 sets of 15 reps.

Step-Up with Bicep Curl:

Stand with your left foot on a strong base or step with 5-pound weights in both hands. With your weight balanced on your left foot, lift yourself so you are standing on the step; raise your right thigh parallel to floor. In the same instance, roll the weights up moving towards the shoulders. Return to your starting position. Do 12 reps, then switch sides and repeat. 3 sets of this exercise are advisable. This exercise works butt, abs, quadriceps, hamstrings, and biceps.

Single-Leg Dumbbell Row:

For this exercise, stand holding a 5 to 10 pound weight in your left hand. Lean forward so an almost parallel to floor back position is created. Place your right hand on a chair in order to develop support for your movement. Stretch the left arm towards the floor with your palm facing in. Lift the left leg straight up behind you, in order for the body to form take the shape of a T. Bend the left elbow and move weight up until the elbow is completely parallel with your torso; stay in this position for 30 seconds, then slowly lower the weight. Do 15 reps, then switch sides and repeat. You can do three sets of this exercise.

Dolphin Plank:

Lie face down with your toes tucked in. Keep your forearms on floor using them as levers, pull your bellybutton in towards your spine using your abs muscles, and make a position of a low plank by raising your hips. Lift your hips further and inhale so body forms an inverted V; pause, and then slowly go back to starting position. Do 4 sets of 10 reps. The Dolphin Plank works on your back, abs, and shoulders.

Superman

Lie face down with arms and legs stretched, with your toes pointed, and your palms down. Raise your arms and legs as high as you can while inhaling; pause, exhale while slowly going back to starting position. Do 4 sets of 10 repeats. This exercise works the back, butt and glutes. While you are trying to build a regimen for weight loss, make sure that you do so in accordance with your health status. Eat enough so that you do not feel too lethargic and are able to maintain an active lifestyle. Keep yourself completely hydrated. Make sure to drink plenty of fluids to get the necessary electrolytes after a workout. Go at your own pace; the weight will drop off if you keep to your routine and diet. Give the new routine a time of at least three weeks before making any changes. You can choose from the variety of exercises stated above. Try and combine a variety of exercises in one session. This allows a maximum amount of targeting in a single session and leaves no area unaddressed. Try and workout for at least three times a week as this allows optimal performance and results. Try to work out a regimen where you can go for a run daily as this is not only beneficial for your weight loss but also helps in overall well-being. It reduces stress and decreases the lethargy. Make sure that you partake in three fulfilling meals a day otherwise you would not have enough energy to go through your day *and* exercise as well. If you feel like snacking try to eat nutritious and energy boosting stuff. Keep your energy up and you will be able to motivate yourself into an active lifestyle that is far more essential to keeping the progress you make in terms of weight loss and sticking to your diet change.

Brian Adams

Chapter 8: Breakfast Recipes

The breakfast the most important meal of the day and therefore you do not skip it under any circumstances. People who do not skip breakfast are actually less likely to be obese or overweight, as they do not tend to indulge in mid-morning sugar cravings. Begin your day with these exciting breakfast recipes that can kick start your vegan journey.

Apple Pancakes:

Ingredients:

- 8 green apples, cored and finely grated

- 1 teaspoon salt

- 6 cups whole wheat pastry flour

- 4 Tablespoons baking powder

- 8 Tablespoons apple juice concentrate, thawed

- Applesauce, to serve

- 3 cups low fat soy milk

Instructions:

1. Take a large bowl. Add the baking powder, salt and flour to it and mix well.
2. In another small bowl, mix the apple juice concentrate and soymilk well.
3. Combine both the wet ingredients and dry ingredients well.
4. Add the finely grated apples to the mixture and mix well.
5. Use cooking spray to grease a non-stick skillet.
6. Pour 3 tablespoons of the batter into the skillet. Spread it and cook it till both sides turn golden brown.
7. Repeat step 6 until you have used up all the batter.
8. Serve the pancakes hot with some applesauce.

Blueberry Oatmeal waffles

Ingredients:

- 6 cups frozen blueberries
- 4 cups white whole wheat flour
- 4 tablespoons baking powder
- 6 cups unsweetened almond milk
- 2 teaspoons salt
- 1 teaspoon ground allspice
- 1 1/3 cups unsweetened applesauce
- 4 cups quick cooking oats
- 8 tablespoons canola oil
- 12 tablespoons pure maple syrup
- 4 teaspoon pure vanilla extract

Instructions:

1. Take a large bowl. Add the baking powder, flour, salt and allspice to it and mix them well.
2. Add the cooked oats to the bowl next and mix well.
3. Create some room in the center of the mixture and add the applesauce, canola oil, almond milk, maple syrup and vanilla.
4. Mix all the ingredients well till it turns into a fine batter.
5. Allow the batter rest for around five minutes in the bowl.
6. Add the frozen blueberries to the batter and combine well.

7. Prepare a waffle iron by brushing it with some oil.

8. Read the instructions on the package of the waffle iron carefully and cook the batter in it.

9. Serve the waffles hot.

Toast with refried beans and avocado

Ingredients:

- 8 slices sandwich bread

- 4 cups homemade vegan refried beans

- 4 avocadoes, thinly sliced

- Coarse sea salt

- A few slivers of white onion

Instructions:

1. First toast your bread slices nicely.
2. As the bread slices are getting toasted, mash the avocadoes separately.
3. Arrange the toasted slices on serving plates.
4. Place the mashed avocado and the refried beans on top of the slices.
5. Arrange the white onions on top of the refried beans.
6. Season the slices with some coarse sea salt and serve hot.

Jelly Filled Muffins

Ingredients:

- 6 cups all-purpose flour

- 2 teaspoons ground nutmeg

- 2 teaspoons baking soda

- 3 teaspoons baking powder

- 4 teaspoons cider vinegar

- 4 cups soy milk

- 2 teaspoons fine salt

- 3 cups + 8 tablespoons granulated sugar

- 8 tablespoons cornstarch

- 1 1/3 cups vegetable oil

- 8 teaspoons vanilla extract

- 1 1/3 cups raspberry jam

- Powdered sugar

Instructions:

1. Preheat the oven to 350 degrees F.

2. Line four muffin pans (12 wells each) with parchment paper.

3. Take a large bowl. Sift the flour into it. Add the baking soda, salt, baking powder and nutmeg to the bowl. Mix all the ingredients well.

4. Take a small bowl. Add the vinegar, soymilk and cornstarch to it and mix well.

5. Mix the flour mixture and the soymilk mixture well.

6. Now add the granulated sugar, vanilla extract and vegetable oil to it and mix well. Make sure there are no lumps while you mix the ingredients together.

7. Now spoon enough batter and fill each muffin cup.

8. Create a small indentation in the middle of each cup and add in the raspberry jam.

9. Place the muffin pans in the oven and bake the muffins for 23 minutes.

10. At the end of 23 minutes, remove the pans from the oven and place them on a wire rack for the muffins to cool.

11. Dust the muffins with the powdered sugar before serving them.

Tofu Breakfast Tacos

Ingredients:

- 4 packages extra-firm tofu
- 8 teaspoons onion powder
- 1 cup whole wheat flour
- 1 cup nutritional yeast
- 8 tablespoons Bragg Liquid Aminos
- 1 teaspoon turmeric
- 2 teaspoons garlic powder
- 32 warmed corn tortillas, to serve
- Salsa, to serve

Instructions:

1. Remove the tofu block from the package and keep it on a plate. Cover the block with another plate and keep some weight on top of it. Allow the tofu block to remain this way for at least 30 minutes. This will allow the excess liquid to drain off from the block. Repeat this process with the other tofu blocks simultaneously.

2. Once the liquid from the tofu blocks have been completely drained off, crumble them finely and transfer it to a bowl.

3. Add the onion powder, garlic powder, wheat flour, turmeric and yeast to the tofu crumble in the bowl. Mix well.

4. Add the liquid aminos to the bowl next and toss all the ingredients.
5. Take a large iron skillet and heat it over medium heat.
6. Transfer the tofu mixture to the skillet. Cook it until the tofu is browned and becomes crisp.
7. Serve it hot with the warm tortillas and salsa.

Vegan Pancakes

Ingredients:

- 2-1/2 cups all-purpose flour
- 1/4 cup white sugar
- 5 teaspoons baking powder
- 1 teaspoon salt
- 2-1/2 cups water
- 2 tablespoons oil

Instructions:

1. In a large bowl sift together the baking powder, flour and salt. In a small bowl, using a whisk, combine the oil and water together.
2. Create a small well in the dry ingredients and slowly pour in the oil and water mixture.
3. Whisk well together; the batter will contain a few lumps.
4. Pour some oil on a griddle and heat over a medium high flame. Pour a large spoon of the batter on the heated griddle and lightly spread it out.
5. Cook until there are bubbles on the batter and edges of the pancake have dried out.
6. Carefully flip the pancake over and cook until the other side is well browned.
7. Repeat with the rest of the batter.

8. Serve with a side of your favorite fruits.

Vegan Spinach and Tofu Quiche

Ingredients:

- 2 cups tofu
- 2/3 cup 1% milk or soy milk
- 1 teaspoon salt, or to taste
- 1 teaspoon pepper
- 2 ½ cups spinach, cut into thin strips
- 2 teaspoons minced garlic
- 1/2 cup diced onion
- 1-1/3 cups Cheddar cheese, shredded
- 1 cup Swiss cheese, shredded
- 2 unbaked 9 inch pie crust

Instructions:

1. Before you start prepping, turn up your oven to about 350 degrees F (175 degrees C) and allow it to preheat.

2. Pour the milk in to a food processor or blender and place the tofu in it. Give it a whirl until it forms a smooth paste; add in some more milk if necessary. Add in the salt and pepper and mix well.

3. Combine the spinach, onion, Swiss cheese, garlic Cheddar cheese and the tofu and milk paste together in a medium sized bowl. Combine well and pour the prepared filling into the unbaked piecrusts.

4. Pop the crust into the preheated oven and bake for about 30 minutes or until the piecrust gets a nice golden brown color.

5. Let the quiche stand for about 5 minutes, before cutting into it and serve hot!

Flax Seed & Pumpkin Loaf

Ingredients:

- 1 tablespoon flax seed meal
- 3 tablespoons water
- 3/4 cup sugar
- 1/2 cup canned pumpkin puree
- 1/4 cup applesauce
- 2/3 cup all-purpose flour
- 8 teaspoons pastry flour (whole wheat)
- 1/2 teaspoon baking soda
- 1/2 teaspoon ground cinnamon
- 1/4 teaspoon salt
- 1/4 teaspoon baking powder
- 1/4 teaspoon ground nutmeg
- 1/8 teaspoon ground cloves

Instructions:

1. Crank up your oven to 350 degrees F (175 degrees C) and allow it to preheat. Lightly spray a 9 x 5 inch loaf pan with some cooking spray.
2. Combine the flax seed meal and water together in a bowl. Whisk well until well blended. Add in the pumpkin puree, sugar and applesauce and mix well.

3. In another large sized bowl, sieve together the all-purpose flour, baking soda, whole wheat flour, cinnamon, baking powder, salt, cloves and nutmeg.

4. Pour this flour mix into the prepared pumpkin and flax seed meal mix and keep stirring until a smooth batter is formed without any lumps.

5. Carefully pour this batter into the greased loaf pan and pop into the preheated oven.

6. Let it bake for about 70 to 75 minutes or until a skewer pricked into the center comes out clean.

7. Remove the loaf from the oven and let it stand for a few minutes before inverting the loaf onto a wire rack.

8. Let the loaf cool a bit before slicing it. Serve the bread warm or store it in an airtight container for later consumption.

Banana, Kale & Soy Milk Smoothie

Ingredients:

- 4 bananas, peeled and chopped into bite sized pieces
- 8 cups kale, chopped
- 2 cups light unsweetened soy milk
- 1/4 cup flax seeds
- 4 teaspoons maple syrup

Instructions:

1. Place the banana and kale in a food processor and blend until it forms a mushy paste.
2. Slowly pour in the soymilk, little by little, and continue blending until it gets a smooth consistency.
3. Add in the flax seeds and maple syrup and whirl until well combined.
4. Fill 4 glasses with a few cubes of ice and divide the smoothie among the four glasses.
5. Serve immediately!

Vegan Crepes

Ingredients:

- 1 cup soy milk
- 1 cup water
- 1/2 cup melted soy margarine
- 2 tablespoons turbinado sugar
- 1/4 cup maple syrup
- 2 cups all-purpose flour
- 1/2 teaspoon salt

Instructions:

1. Combine the soymilk, turbinado sugar, all-purpose flour, soy margarine, maple syrup, water and salt in a large mixing bowl. Cover this mixture with a plastic wrap and leave it aside for about 2 hours.

2. Spray a 6 inch skillet with some cooking spray or grease it with some soy margarine. Place the skillet on a high flame and heat until the skillet is hot.

3. Spoon out the prepared batter onto the skillet, about 3 tablespoons at a time and move the skillet around so that the batter covers the bottom of the skillet.

4. Once a side is browned, flip it over and cook the other side until it is well browned.

5. Serve with a side of freshly cut fruit.

Poppy and Lemon Scones

Ingredients:

- 2 cups flour
- ¾ cups sugar
- ½ cup soy milk
- ½ cup water
- 4 tea spoons baking powder
- ½ tea spoon salt
- ¾ cup soy margarine
- 1 lemon, juiced and zested
- 2 table spoons poppy seeds

Instructions:

1. Preheat your oven to 400 degrees Fahrenheit (200 degrees Celsius).
2. Grease a baking sheet.
3. Add the sugar, flour, baking powder and salt into a large bowl. Use a sifter to prevent any lumps. Add to this the soy margarine in pieces and continue rubbing it in. Doing this manually will help remove lumps and rub the margarine into the flour using your hands. It yields better results. Continue this process until the mixture resembles granulated sand.

4. Stir into the mixture the lemon zest, poppy seeds, and the lemon juice.

5. Dilute the soymilk with the water in the ingredient list. Slowly stir this combination into the dry ingredients until the batter turns wet, and should have biscuit dough consistency. Add the liquid only as required because not all of it may be needed in the end.

6. Now using a spoon drop lumps of the batter on to the greased baking sheet. Try making them about three inches apart from each other so they have room to expand.

7. In the preheated oven, bake them for about 10 to 15 minute, until they turn golden.

Simple Home-style Potato Pancakes

Ingredients:

- 10 potatoes (peel and shred them)
- 1 onion chopped finely
- 1 carrot peeled and finely shredded.
- 6 cloves of garlic, crushed
- 1 table spoon finely chopped fresh coriander
- 1 table spoon finely chopped fresh dill
- 2 table spoons of fresh squeezed lemon juice
- 2 table spoons of all-purpose plain flour
- ¼ cup olive oil
- 2 cups of bread crumbs
- Salt to taste
- Pepper to taste
- Oil for frying, as required (you can use canola or olive)

Instructions:

1. Combine the potatoes, onion, carrot, garlic, coriander, and the dill in a large bowl.
2. Mix in the lemon juice, the 1/4 cup of olive oil, breadcrumbs, plain flour, salt, and pepper. Knead this mixture gently just until it holds together.

3. Heat the frying oil in a skillet over a medium heat. Drop dollops of the mixture into the hot oil and try not to crowd the pan. Cook for approximately 4 minutes per side, or until golden brown. Serve hot. Enjoy!

Chapter 9: Soup Recipes

Soups are a delicious combination of flavors and textures in one bowl! Begin your meal with some deliciousness by following some of these vegan soup recipes.

Delicious Peanut & Sweet Potato Soup

Ingredients:
- 2 tablespoons vegetable oil
- 2 large onions, chopped
- 4 cloves of garlic, minced
- 4 teaspoons fresh ginger root, minced
- 1 tablespoon ground cumin
- 1 tablespoon ground coriander seeds
- 1 teaspoon ground cinnamon
- 2 pinches ground cloves

- 6 medium tomatoes, chopped
- 3 pounds sweet potatoes, rinsed, peeled and chopped
- 2 carrot, peeled and chopped
- 9 cups water
- 2 teaspoons salt
- 1/2 cup dry-roasted peanuts, unsalted and chopped
- 2 pinches cayenne pepper
- 1/4 cup creamy peanut butter
- 2 bunches chopped fresh cilantro

Instructions:

1. Place a medium sized saucepan on a medium high flame. Pour in the oil and heat it. Once the oil is hot, add in the onions and sauté for about 10 minutes or until the onions are lightly caramelized. Add in the ginger, garlic, coriander seeds, cumin, cloves and cinnamon to the pan and mix well. Fry lightly until the aroma of the spices fills the kitchen.

2. Add the sweet potatoes, tomatoes and carrots to the pan and continue cooking for about 5 more minutes. Constantly stir the vegetables while they cook.

3. Pour the water into the pan and season the soup with salt according to taste. Once the soup starts boiling, reduce the

flame and let the soup simmer for about 30 minutes on a low flame.

4. Take the saucepan off the heat and pour it into a blender or a food processor. Add in the peanuts and whirl until a smooth concoction is formed. Add in some cayenne pepper and pour the contents of the blender into a saucepan.

5. Add in the peanut butter and heat on a medium low flame until the soup is well heated through. Do not let the soup boil.

6. Serve hot garnished with some fresh cilantro.

Red Lentil and Butternut Squash Soup

Ingredients:

- 2 tablespoons peanut oil
- 1 large onion, chopped
- 2 tablespoons fresh ginger root, minced
- 2 cloves of garlic, chopped finely
- 2 pinches fenugreek seeds
- 2 cups dry red lentils
- 2 cups butternut squash - skinned, seeded, and cubed
- 2/3 cup fresh cilantro, finely chopped
- 4 cups water
- 2 cups coconut milk
- 1/4 cup tomato paste
- 2 teaspoons curry powder
- 2 pinches cayenne pepper
- 2 pinches ground nutmeg
- Salt, to taste
- Pepper, to taste

Instructions:

1. Pour the oil into a large sized pot and heat over a medium flame. Once the oil is hot, add the onion, garlic, ginger and fenugreek to the pot and cook until the onions turn translucent and soft.

2. Add the lentils, cilantro and squash into the pot and mix with a light hand. Pour in the water, tomato paste and coconut milk into the pot and stir well.

3. Taste and season with cayenne pepper, curry powder, nutmeg, pepper and salt. Increase or decrease the quantities of the spices as required.

4. Heat the soup until it is bubbling. Reduce the flame and let the soup simmer for about half an hour or until the squash and lentils have become soft and tender.

5. Serve hot!

Black Bean & Corn Kernel Soup

Ingredients:

- 2 tablespoons olive oil
- 2 large onions, chopped
- 2 stalks of celery, chopped
- 4 carrots, peeled and chopped
- 8 cloves garlic, chopped
- 1/4 cup chili powder
- 2 tablespoons ground cumin
- 2 pinches black pepper
- 8 cups vegetable broth
- 8 (15 ounce) cans black beans
- 2 (15 ounce) cans whole kernel corn
- 2 (14.5 ounce) cans crushed tomatoes

Instructions:

1. Pour the oil into a large sized pot and heat over a medium high flame. Once the oil is heated, add in the onion, carrots, celery and garlic and sauté for about 5 minutes.
2. Season the soup with cumin, chili powder and black pepper. Cook the soup for another minute, before adding in the vegetable broth, 4 cans of corn kernels and 4 cans of black beans.
3. Heat the pot until the soup starts bubbling.

4. Add the remaining 4 cans of corn kernels, 4 cans of black beans and tomatoes into a blender or food processor whirl until it forms a smooth paste.

5. Pour the paste into the bubbling soup and mix well.

6. Reduce the heat and let the soup simmer for another 15 minutes.

7. Serve hot

Vegan Style Hot and Sour Soup

Ingredients:

- 2 ounces dried wood ear mushrooms
- 8 dried shiitake mushrooms
- 24 dried tiger lily buds
- 4 cups hot water
- 1/2 ounce bamboo fungus
- 6 tablespoons soy sauce
- 10 tablespoons rice vinegar
- 1/2 cup cornstarch
- 2 cups firm tofu, cut into strips ¼ inch thick
- 8 cups vegetable broth
- 1/2 teaspoon crushed red pepper flakes
- 1 teaspoon ground black pepper
- 1-1/2 teaspoons ground white pepper
- 1 tablespoon chili oil
- 1 tablespoon sesame oil
- 2 green onion, sliced
- 2 cups Chinese dried mushrooms

Instructions:

1. Place the dried wood ear mushrooms, tiger lily buds, and shiitake mushrooms in a bowl and cover with about 3 cups

of hot water. Let the mushrooms and buds soak in the hot water for about 20 minutes, or until they get rehydrated.

2. Drain the water and save the water for later. Remove the stems from the mushrooms and chop into thin strips. Chop the tiger lily buds in half. Save the liquid.

3. In another bowl, place the bamboo fungus and cover with ½ cup lightly heated and salted water. Let the bamboo fungus soak for about 20 minutes until it gets rehydrated. Drain the water (and save it) and mince the bamboo fungus finely.

4. Whisk together the rice vinegar, 2 tablespoons cornstarch and soy sauce in a third small bowl. Place about half of the prepared tofu strips in the mixture and let them soak.

5. Combine the vegetables broth and the saved tiger lily bud liquid and the mushroom liquid in a large saucepan and heat over a medium flame. When the liquid starts bubbling, add in the rehydrated tiger lily buds, shiitake mushrooms and the wood mushrooms and mix well.

6. Reduce the heat and let the liquid simmer for another 5 to 7 minutes. Add in the black pepper, red pepper and white pepper and stir.

7. Combine the remaining cornstarch and the bamboo fungus water in a small bowl. Mix well until the cornstarch

dissolves and pour it into the saucepan containing the soup. Mix well until the soup thickens.

8. Pour the prepared soy mix and the remaining tofu strips into the soup. Turn up the heat and bring the soup to a boil. Add in the chili oil, bamboo fungus and sesame oil to the soup and mix lightly.

9. Serve hot topped with some green onion!

Delicious Black and White Bean Soup

Ingredients:

- 2 tablespoons olive oil
- 1 large onion, chopped
- 2 celery ribs, chopped
- 2 tablespoons garlic, crushed
- 2 teaspoons thyme
- 2 (14.5 ounce) cans black beans, drained
- 16 cups vegetable broth, divided
- 2 teaspoons ground cumin
- 2 (14.5 ounce) cans white beans, drained
- 1 teaspoon dried sage

Instructions:

1. Pour the oil into a large pot and heat over a medium flame. Once the oil is hot, add in it the onion, garlic, celery and thyme to it and cook for about 10 to 12 minutes or until the celery gets tender.
2. Add the black beans, cumin and 8 cups of vegetable broth to the pot and mix well.
3. Add in the white beans, the remaining 8 cups of vegetable broth and the sage into the pot and mix well.

4. Turn up the heat and heat the pot till the soup starts bubbling. Immediately lower the flame and let the soup simmer on a low flame for about 30 to 45 minutes.

5. Serve hot!

Vegan Borscht

Ingredients:

- 1-1/2 teaspoons olive oil
- 1-1/2 cloves garlic, minced
- 1 small onion, chopped
- 6 1/2 teaspoons olive oil
- 1 stalk celery, chopped
- 2 small carrots, finely chopped
- 1/2 green bell pepper, chopped
- 1 large beet, including greens, diced
- 1/2 (16 ounce) can whole peeled tomatoes
- 1/4 cup canned peeled and diced tomatoes
- 1 potato, quartered
- 1/2 cup Swiss chard, shredded
- 1 cup vegetable broth
- 2 cups water
- 1 tablespoon dill weed
- Freshly ground pepper,
- Salt, to taste
- 1 cup silken tofu

Instructions:

1. Pour the 1 ½ teaspoons olive oil into a large skillet and heat over a medium flame. Once the oil is hot, add in the onion and garlic. Keep cooking until the onion gets tender and translucent, this should take about 5 to 7 minutes. Keep aside.

2. In a large pot, add the remaining 6 ½ teaspoons of olive oil over a medium high flame. Add in the celery, bell pepper, whole tomatoes, Swiss chard, carrots, beets with the greens, diced tomatoes, the onion and garlic mixture, and potatoes and mix well. Keep cooking until the Swiss chard lightly wilts; this will take about 5 to 10 minutes.

3. Once the chard is wilted around the edges, immediately add the water, vegetable broth and dill weed to the pot. Season with salt and pepper according to taste.

4. Once the soup comes to a boil, reduce the heat to a low flame and let the soup simmer for about an hour.

5. Strain about half the beets from the soup and place in a blender. Do not fill more than half of the jar. Hold the lid of the jar down using a folded towel and start blending the beets. First with a few short pulses and then leave it on until the beets are pureed.

6. Add in the silken tofu and blend until smooth. Pour the beet and tofu paste into the soup pot. Keep simmering the

soup until it reduces by a third; this will take another hour on a low flame.

7. This soup can be served either hot or cold!

Delicious Vegan Style Corn Chowder

Ingredients:

- 1/4 cup olive oil
- 1 large onion, chopped
- 2 cups celery, chopped
- 2 cups carrots, chopped
- 2 cloves garlic, minced
- 5 cups water
- 4 cubes vegetable bouillon
- 4 cups corn
- 4 cups soy milk
- 2 tablespoons flour
- 2 teaspoons dried parsley
- 2 teaspoons garlic powder
- 2 teaspoons salt
- 2 teaspoons pepper

Instructions:

1. Pour the oil into a large skillet and heat over a medium flame. Once the oil is hot, add in the onion and celery and cook until the onion is slightly caramelized. Add in the carrots and garlic to the skillet and keep cooking until the garlic gets a light golden hue.

2. In a large pot, pour the water and heat it over a high flame until the water boils. Add in the bouillon cubes and reduce the heat to a medium low flame. Once the bouillon cubes have dissolved in the water, add in the vegetables from the skillet and corn to the pot.

3. Keep cooking until the vegetables are soft and tender. If you feel that the liquid is running out, add in some more water to the pot.

4. Further reduce the heat to a low flame and add in about 2cups of the soymilk to the pot. Keep mixing well and add the leftover 2 cups of soymilk.

5. Slowly add in the flour, constantly stirring it to ensure that there are no lumps formed. Add in the garlic powder and parsley. Mix well. Taste and season accordingly with salt and pepper.

6. Keep simmering the chowder over a low flame until it thickens; this will take about 15 to 20 minutes.

7. Serve hot!

Brian Adams

Chapter 10: Main Course Recipes

In this chapter, we present to you some exciting main course recipes that will not only satiate your hunger, but also satiate your need for some much needed nutrients. Help yourselves.

Special Vegan Kofte

Ingredients:
- 2 x 400 g tin of chickpeas, rinsed drained
- 2 teaspoons cumin seeds
- 80 g fine breadcrumbs
- 2 teaspoons coriander seeds
- 2 pieces of fresh ginger, finely chopped
- 4 courgettes
- 4 cloves of garlic, finely chopped
- olive oil

- 2 large bunches of fresh coriander
- freshly ground black pepper
- fine sea salt

For the minty yoghurt dip:
- 1 cucumber, deseeded and chopped roughly
- 8 tablespoons soya yoghurt
- 6 sprigs of fresh mint, finely chopped
- Juice from 2 lemons

For the nutty sauce:

- 200 g cashew nuts
- 280 ml light coconut milk
- 2 cloves of garlic, peeled and chopped
- 2 small onions, peeled and chopped
- 4 tablespoons smooth peanut butter

Instructions:
1. Take a small frying pan. Toast the coriander and the cumin seeds in the pan over medium heat.
2. Remove the pan from the heat and transfer its contents to a mortar. Powder the toasted coriander and cumin seeds in the mortar.
3. Add the finely chopped ginger and garlic to a frying pan. Pour some oil into the pan and fry it for around 3 minutes

till the garlic turns golden brown. Transfer the garlic and ginger to a food processor.

4. Finely grate the courgettes next. Place the coriander on them and season with the salt.

5. Squeeze the mixture well using your hands to drain off any excess fluid. Transfer the courgette mixture to the food processor.

6. Separate the coriander leaves from their stalks and keep them aside.

7. Place half the coriander stalks in the food processor.

8. Add the chickpeas, breadcrumbs, pepper and salt to the food processor.

9. Pulse the contents of the food processor well till the mixture reaches a smooth consistency.

10. Transfer the mixture to a clean tray and shape them into 16 little fingers. Place the tray in the refrigerator for around twenty minutes.

11. Take a small bowl. Add the chopped cucumber, yogurt and mint leaves to it. Pour the lemon juice over it and mix well.

12. Slice the remainder of the coriander stalks finely.

13. Take a large frying pan and add some oil to it. Add the chopped coriander stalks, garlic and onions to it and fry it over medium heat.

14. Add the cashews to the pan and fry them for around two minutes.

15. Transfer the contents of the frying pan to a food processor. Add the coconut milk and peanut butter to the food processor. Pulse the contents of the food processor till it reaches a thick consistency.

16. Pour some oil into a large frying pan and fry the Kofte in it, one at a time.

17. Serve them hot with the nutty sauce and the yogurt dip.

Chili Con Veggie

Ingredients:

- 4 x400 grams tins of red kidney beans, drained and rinsed
- 2.4 liters of organic vegetable stock
- 8 cloves of garlic, peeled and chopped finely
- 4 medium onions, peeled and chopped finely
- 2 medium leeks, trimmed and chopped finely
- 2 long fresh red chilies, deseeded and chopped finely
- 4 tablespoons smoked paprika
- 2 whole nutmeg, for grating
- 4 tablespoons ground cumin
- 4 tablespoons ground coriander
- 1 cinnamon stick
- 4 tablespoons tomato purée
- 500 g dried green lentils
- 4 tablespoons dried oregano
- 500 g dried red lentils
- 4x 400 grams tins of black beans, drained and rinsed
- 4x 400 grams tins of chopped tomatoes
- 4 tablespoons olive oil
- sea salt
- freshly ground black pepper
- Rice, to serve

Instructions:

1. Take a heavy bottomed pan and pour some oil into it. Add the chopped leeks, onions, chili and garlic to the pan and fry it over medium heat. Fry them till they turn soft.

2. Add the spices, dried herbs and nutmeg to the pan and fry for another two minutes.

3. Add the tomato puree to the pan and cook for another two minutes.

4. Add the chopped tomatoes, lentils and beans to the pan.

5. Pour the vegetable stock into the pan and bring the mixture to a boil. Season with salt and pepper.

6. Allow the mixture to simmer for another hour till the mixture thickens.

7. Serve the curry hot with rice.

Beetroot Carpaccio

Ingredients:

- 16 medium beetroots
- Juice and zest from 4 lemons
- 2 tablespoons capers, drained and rinsed
- 2 red onions, finely chopped
- 4 teaspoons caster sugar
- 4 tablespoons olive oil
- a small bunch of fresh dill, finely chopped
- Water

Instructions:

1. Take a large saucepan and fill it with water. Place the beets in the water and bring it to a boil.
2. Allow it to simmer for around forty minutes. At the end of 40 minutes, drain the water and keep the cooked beets aside.
3. Take a small bowl. Add the lemon juice, zest, dill, onion, olive oil, sugar, salt and capers to it and mix well.
4. Run the cooked beets under cold water and peel their skins. Slice the beets thinly.
5. Place the thin slices of beets on a large plate. Pour the dressing over each slice.

6. Cover the plate with some foil and place it in the refrigerator for around two hours.

7. Serve cold.

Vegetable Curry

Ingredients:
- 2400 ml curry base sauce
- 2 butternut squash, peeled and diced
- 400 g mushrooms, cut into quarters
- 4 courgettes, diced
- 4 medium red onions, peeled and chopped
- 4 red peppers, diced
- 600 g cauliflower, broken into florets
- Water
- vegetable oil

Instructions:
1. Take a large frying pan and pour some vegetable oil into it.
2. Add the chopped onions to the pan and fry it for ten minutes till they turn golden brown.
3. Add the chopped vegetables into the pan, one at a time. Mix well.
4. Pour the curry base sauce into the pan. Combine all the ingredients well.
5. Allow the mixture to simmer for around 30 minutes for the curry to reach a thick consistency. Pour some water if the curry becomes too thick.
6. Serve the curry hot.

Brian Adams

Vegan Burger

Ingredients:

- 4 whole meal burger buns
- 2 large ripe tomatoes, cut into thin slices
- 3 heaped tablespoons plain flour
- 340 g of sweet corn
- 400 g of chickpeas, drained and rinsed
- ½ teaspoon coriander powder
- ½ teaspoon paprika
- ½ teaspoon cumin powder
- sea salt
- zest of a lemon
- rapeseed oil
- 1 medium lettuce, washed
- Half a bunch of fresh coriander
- tomato ketchup

Instructions:

1. Add the sweet corn and chickpeas to a food processor.
2. Separate the coriander leaves from their stalks and keep them aside.
3. Place half the coriander stalks and leaves in the food processor.

4. Mix the spices, flour, lemon zest, and salt to the food processor.

5. Pulse the contents of the food processor until well combined.

6. Shape the mixture into 4 evenly sized patties. Place the patties on a tray and refrigerate for 30 minutes.

7. Take some oil in a large frying pan. Fry the patties in the pan over medium heat for ten minutes until browned.

8. Spread some ketchup on the base of each bun.

9. Arrange a few slices of tomato, lettuce, coriander leaves and fried patty on top of the bun. Top it with the other bun. Serve immediately.

Chunky Vegan Chili

Ingredients:

- 1 cup brown lentils, soak it overnight
- 1 cup kidney beans, soak it overnight
- 1 cup white beans, soak it overnight 12 cups water
- 12 cups chopped fresh tomatoes
- 1 cup chopped green bell pepper
- 2 cups chopped fresh mushrooms
- 1 cup fresh green beans
- 1 cup chopped red bell pepper
- 1 cup chopped celery
- 1 small red onion, chopped
- 1 small onion, chopped
- 1-1/2 cups tofu, crumbled
- Black pepper,
- Salt, to taste
- Onion powder, as per taste
- Chili powder, as per taste
- Garlic powder, as per taste

Instructions:

1. Drain the water from the lentils, kidney beans and white beans and rinse them well. Pour all the beans in a large pot

and add enough water just to cover the beans. Heat the pot on a medium high flame for at least an hour, or until the beans are tender.

2. While the beans boil, place a large saucepan on a high flame. Put the water and tomatoes in the saucepan and bring the mixture to a boil. Reduce the flame and let the tomatoes simmer for an hour without any cover or until the tomatoes break down.

3. Pour the contents of the saucepan into the pot and mix well. Add the green bell pepper, green beans, onion, mushrooms, red bell pepper, celery and tofu into the pot.

4. Taste and add the seasonings accordingly.

5. Simmer the chili for another 3 hours or until it reaches the consistency required.

6. Serve hot!

Fiery Potato & Chickpea Curry

Ingredients:

- 8 potatoes, peeled and cubed
- 1/4 cup vegetable oil
- 1 large yellow onion, diced
- 6 cloves garlic, minced
- 4 teaspoons ground cumin
- 1 tablespoon cayenne pepper
- 8 teaspoons curry powder
- 8 teaspoons garam masala (spice blend, available in most supermarkets Indian stores)
- 2 (1 inch) pieces of fresh ginger root, peeled and minced
- 4 teaspoons salt
- 4 cups tomatoes, diced
- 4 cups garbanzo beans (chickpeas), soaked overnight, drained and rinsed
- 4 cups peas
- 4 cups coconut milk

Instructions:

1. Pour water into a large pot and add some salt to it. Bring the water to a boil and add in the potatoes. Reduce the heat to a medium low flame, cover the pot and let it simmer for about 15 minutes or until the potatoes are tender.

2. Drain the potatoes from the liquid and let the potatoes steam dry for a few minutes.

3. Pour the vegetable oil into a large skillet and heat over a medium flame. Add in the garlic and onion and keep cooking until the onion turns translucent and softens; this should take about 7 minutes.

4. Season the onion with cayenne pepper, cumin, garam masala, curry powder, salt and ginger. Cook for another 2 minutes or till the spices get aromatic.

5. Add the garbanzo beans, tomatoes, potatoes and peas to the skillet and mix well.

6. Pour the coconut milk in to the skillet and let the liquid simmer for about 10 minutes.

7. Serve hot with a side of *naan* (Indian flat bread) or over a bed of steamed rice.

Chapter 11: Side Dish Recipes

The duty of the side dish is not to overshadow a main dish, rather to complement it and provide the eater a break from the monotony of the main dish. In this chapter you will find a list of such delicious and enticing side dishes that will leave you licking your lips!

Vegan Agedashi Tofu

Ingredients:

- 3 cups extra firm tofu
- 6 tablespoons cornstarch
- Oil, for frying
- 2 large green onions, chopped
- 1/4 cup hoisin sauce

Instructions:

1. Cut the tofu into about 24 cubes. Pour the cornstarch in a shallow dish with raised sides. Place the tofu cubes in the cornstarch and lightly shake the dish so that the tofu cubes get a thin and even coating of cornstarch on them.

2. Pour enough oil into a skillet to cover half the tofu cubes and heat the oil on a high flame. Once heated through, lower the flame to a medium low and gently fry the tofu cubes for about 4 minutes on each side or until the tofu cube is golden brown and crispy.

3. Remove the done tofu cubes and place on an absorbent sheet.

4. Toss the green onions over the fried tofu cubes and spoon the hoisin sauce over the tofu and onions. Immediately serve he dish without delay.

Mediterranean Style Vegan Couscous

Ingredients:

- 2-1/2 cups vegetable broth
- 2-1/2 cups water
- 4 cups pearl (Israeli) couscous
- 2 pinches salt
- 2 pinches ground black pepper
- 10 tablespoons olive oil, divided
- 1 cup pine nuts
- 8 cloves of garlic, minced
- 2 shallots, minced
- 1 cup sliced black olives
- 2/3 cup sun-dried tomatoes packed in oil, drained and chopped
- 2 cups vegetable broth
- 1/2 cup chopped fresh flat-leaf parsley

Instructions:

1. Pour the vegetable broth and water into a large saucepan and heat on a high flame, till the mixture starts boiling. Then add in the couscous and sprinkle salt and pepper. Reduce the flame to about medium low and let the mix simmer until the couscous absorbs all the liquid; this will take about 10 minutes.

2. In another skillet, pour 6 tablespoons of olive oil and heat over a medium high flame. Add in the pine nuts and lightly fry them until the aroma of toasted pine nuts fills the kitchen and the nuts get a nice toasted golden brown look. This will take about 1 minute. Take the skillet off heat.

3. Pour the remaining 4 tablespoons olive oil into a saucepan and heat on a medium high flame. Add in the garlic and shallots and cook until they are tender. This should take about 2 minutes.

4. Add in the sun dried tomatoes and black olives into the shallot and garlic mix and cook until they are well heated. Slowly pour the 2 cups vegetable broth and heat until it is bubbling. Reduce the flame to medium low and let the sauce simmer for about 10 minutes to reduce the sauce.

5. Pour the prepared couscous into a large bowl and pour the prepared sauce on the couscous. Mix well and serve garnished with some chopped parsley and the toasted pine nuts.

Sweet & Spicy Vegan Baked Beans

Ingredients:

- 1 cup dry navy beans
- 3 cups water
- 1 tablespoon olive oil
- 1 cup chopped sweet onions
- 1 small clove of garlic, minced
- 2 cups tomato sauce
- 2 tablespoons firmly packed brown sugar
- 2 tablespoons molasses
- 1 tablespoon cider vinegar
- 1-1/2 bay leaves
- 1/2 teaspoon dry mustard
- 1/8 teaspoon ground black pepper
- 1/8 teaspoon ground nutmeg
- 1/8 teaspoon ground cinnamon

Instructions:

1. Pour the water into a large pot and bring to a boil over a high flame. Carefully add the dried navy beans to the pot and reduce the flame to a medium low flame. Continue cooking the beans for an hour or until the beans are soft but firm, occasionally stirring them.

2. Drain the water from the beans and place the beans in a large casserole dish.

3. Crank up your oven to 300 degrees F (150 degrees C) and let it preheat for at least 10 minutes.

4. Pour the olive oil into a skillet and heat over a medium high flame. Add in the onions and cook them until they are translucent and tender. Add the contents of the skillet to the casserole dish and mix well. Pour the tomato sauce over the beans and onion – garlic mixture and stir well.

5. Add in the garlic and cook until caramelized. Add in the brown sugar, cider vinegar, dry mustard, ground nutmeg, molasses, bay leaves, ground black pepper and ground cinnamon and mix well.

6. Cover the casserole dish with a layer of aluminum foil and pop into the preheated oven.

7. Bake for about 3 and half hours, stirring at regular intervals. Add water if you feel the dish is getting too dry.

8. After 3 and half hours have ended, remove the aluminum foil and bake for another 30 minutes without any cover.

9. Serve hot!

Spicy Sweet Potato Sticks

Ingredients:

- 2 tablespoons olive oil
- 1 teaspoon paprika
- 16 sweet potatoes

Instructions:

1. Crank up your oven to 400 degrees F (200 degrees C) and allow preheating for about 10 minutes. Grease a baking sheet with some oil or spray with cooking spray.

2. Wash the sweet potatoes under running water and scrub off the dirt. Cut the sweet potatoes into ½ inch sticks lengthwise.

3. Combine the oil and paprika in a large bowl. Add in the prepared potato sticks and toss well with your hands, ensuring that a layer of the paprika oil coats each potato stick.

4. Place the potato sticks separately on the greased baking sheet in a single line. Ensure that the potato sticks do not overlap each other.

5. Pop the baking sheet into the preheated oven and bake for about 40 minutes.

6. Remove the baking sheet from the oven and let it cool completely before serving.

Brian Adams

Spicy Vegan Style Curried Rice

Ingredients:

- 1/4 cup olive oil
- 2 tablespoons minced garlic
- Black pepper, to taste
- 2 tablespoons ground cumin, or to taste
- 2 tablespoons ground curry powder, or to taste
- 2 tablespoons chili powder, or to taste
- 2 cubes vegetable bouillon
- 2 cups water
- 2 tablespoons soy sauce
- 2 cups uncooked white rice

Instructions:

1. Pour the olive oil in a medium sized saucepan and heat over a low flame. Lightly fry the garlic until its aroma fills the kitchen. Add in the black pepper, curry powder, cumin and chili powder to the saucepan and mix well.
2. Once the spices become aromatic, add in the bouillon cube and add a little water to it. Mix well.
3. Increase the flame to high heat and pour in the remaining water and soy sauce. Add the rice to the saucepan just before the mixture starts boiling and mix well.

4. Once the mixture starts bubbling, lower the flame and cover the pan with a lid. Let the contents of the saucepan simmer for about 20 to 25 minutes or until the rice absorbs all the liquid.

5. Take the saucepan off heat and it stand covered for 5 minutes.

6. Serve hot!

Vegan Tomato & Chili Refried Beans

Ingredients:

- 2 tablespoons olive oil
- 2 onion, diced
- 4 cups pinto beans, soaked overnight and drained
- 3 tablespoons tomato paste
- Chili powder to taste
- 2 cups vegetable broth

Instructions:

1. Pour the oil into a medium sized skillet and heat over a medium flame. Add the onions to the hot oil and sauté until the onion turns translucent and tender.
2. Add in the beans, chili powder, tomato paste and vegetable broth into the skillet. Cook the beans until they are tender and the stock has reduced.
3. Using a potato masher, mash the beans.
4. Serve hot!

Baked Sugar Snap Peas

Ingredients:

- 1 pound sugar snap peas
- kosher salt as per taste
- 2 tablespoons olive oil
- 2 tablespoons shallots, chopped
- 2 teaspoons chopped fresh thyme,

Instructions:

1. Crank up your oven to 450 degrees F (230 degrees C) and let it preheat for about 10 to 20 minutes.
2. On a baking sheet, spread the sugar snap peas in a single layer. Using a pastry brush, lightly dab some olive oil on the sugar snap peas.
3. Sprinkle the chopped shallots, chopped thyme and the kosher salt over the oiled sugar snap peas.
4. Pop the baking sheet into the preheated oven and bake for about 8 minutes or until the
5. Sugar snap peas are soft, yet firm.
6. Serve hot!

Cheesy Potato au Gratin

Ingredients:

- 12 large potatoes, peeled and cubed
- 2-1/2 cups vegetable broth, divided
- 1/4 cup all-purpose flour
- 2 teaspoons seasoning salt
- 1 teaspoon ground black pepper
- 1/2 teaspoon dry mustard
- 1/4 teaspoon nutmeg
- 4 cups soy milk
- 3 cups Cheddar-flavored soy cheese, shredded
- 2 cups bread crumbs
- 2 tablespoons paprika

Instructions:

1. Crank up your oven to 350 degrees F and let it preheat.
2. Pour water into a large pot, add some salt to it and bring it to a boil. Add the potatoes to the salt water and let them cook for about 15 minutes or until they are tender but firm.
3. Drain the water from the potatoes and place them in a 13 x 9 inch baking dish.
4. Pour about 4 tablespoons of the broth into a saucepan and bring to a boil over a high flame. Reduce the heat and add in the flour, salt, mustard, nutmeg and pepper. Mix well.

5. Slowly pour the soy milk into the saucepan and cook, stirring constantly, until the mixture thickens. Add in half of the soy cheese and keep stirring it until the cheese has completely melted. Pour the prepared sauce over the potatoes in the baking dish.

6. Combine remaining broth and the breadcrumbs together in a small bowl. Pour this mix over the sauce covered potatoes. Add in the remaining soy cheese. Lightly top with the paprika.

7. Pop into the preheated oven and bake for about 20 to 25 minutes. Remove from oven and let it stand or about 5 minutes before serving.

8. Serve hot!

Baked Garlicky Potatoes & Mushrooms

Ingredients:

- 2 pounds new potatoes, cut into halves
- 1/4 cup olive oil
- 1 pound Portobello mushrooms
- 12 cloves unpeeled garlic
- 1/4 cup fresh thyme, chopped
- 2 tablespoons olive oil
- kosher salt, as per taste
- ground black pepper, to taste
- 1/2 pound cherry tomatoes
- 1/4 cup toasted pine nuts
- 1/2 pound spinach, thinly sliced

Instructions:

1. Turn up your oven to 425 degrees F (220 degrees C) and let it preheat for some time.

2. In a shallow baking pan, place the new potatoes and sprinkle 4 tablespoons of olive oil over them. Let the potatoes roast in the preheated oven for about 20 minutes, turning them over around the 10 minute mark.

3. Add in the Portobello mushrooms and place them with their stem side up. Also add in the garlic cloves. Lightly sprinkle the chopped thyme on the vegetables and drizzle

the 2 tablespoon olive oil over them. Season to taste with the salt and pepper. Return the baking pan to the oven and bake for another 5 minutes.

4. Remove the baking pan from the oven and add in the cherry tomatoes. Pop the baking pan back into the oven and cook for another 5 minutes, or until the mushrooms soften.

5. Top with the toasted pine nuts and serve with a side of the sliced spinach.

Quick & Easy Cauliflower & Carrot Farro

Ingredients:

- 3 cups farro
- 1/4 cup olive oil
- 2 heads cauliflower, broken into small florets
- 1 large onion, diced
- 1 large carrot, diced
- 1 large celery stalk, diced
- Salt, to taste
- 1/4 cup fresh lemon juice

Instructions:

1. Pour water into a large pot, add in some salt and heat over a high flame until it starts to boil. Add in the faro and keep

heating the pot until the farro is tender. This should take about 30 minutes. Drain the water from the farro and set the farro aside.

2. While the farro is cooking, pour the olive oil into a large skillet and heat over a medium flame. Add the onion and cauliflower to the skillet and cook until the onion gets translucent and the cauliflower starts to soften. This will take about 10 to 12 minutes.

3. Add in the chopped carrot, celery stem and salt to the skillet with the cauliflower and onion and mix well. Keep stirring the mix and keep cooking until the cauliflower is completely soft.

4. Mix the vegetable mixture and the prepared farro together in a large mixing bowl. Pour the lemon juice over the vegetable and farro mixture and stir well.

5. Serve immediately.

Brian Adams

Chapter 12: Salads

On the offset one assumes that vegan diet is composed entirely of variations of salads. But as the amazing variety of dishes given in this book show, vegan diet is complex and delicious to boot. Salads are however an integral part of maintaining a well-balanced diet as they can be developed in a variety of ways and nearly always help you in managing your essential diet requirements of the day. Salads can practically be developed with *anything* that you might have in the fridge, just be sure to add a nice serving of fruit or vegetables. Here are some recipes for salads that are fulfilling and make for a nice light lunch on their own if you are on a diet.

Summer Brown Rice Salad with Dried Nuts:

Ingredients:

- 1 cup of brown rice
- ¾ cup frozen peas
- 1 pear diced into ½ inch pieces
- ¼ cup dried cherries, roughly chopped
- 1/3 cup cashews roughly chopped
- 1 bunch of chives finely chopped

For the dressing

- 2 cloves of garlic, minced
- 1 table spoon maple syrup
- 1 tea spoon soy sauce
- 1 tea spoon tahini sauce
- 2 table spoons olive oil
- 2 table spoons balsamic vinegar
- 4 table spoons toasted sesame or flax seeds

Instructions:

1. Cook the rice in about three cups of water till cooked through.
2. Fluff and set aside, cooling them to room temperature.
3. Flash boil the peas until tender.
4. Combine the peas, pear, cherries, cashews and chives with the cooled rice in a large bowl.

5. Combine all the ingredients for the dressing and whisk until completely amalgamated.

6. Stir the dressing into the rice mixture until it coats all the ingredients.

7. Dress with extra chives and sesame or flax seeds.

8. Leave in the refrigerator for a few hours if possible, this enhances the flavors.

Citrusy Quinoa Salad

Ingredients:

- 1 cup quinoa, uncooked and rinsed and drained
- 2 cups of water
- 2 oranges (juicy and large)
- ¼ cup olive oil
- 2 tea spoons vinegar (try apple cider)
- ½ tea spoon honey or maple syrup
- ½ tea spoon toasted coriander seeds, crush slightly to enhance flavor
- Salt to taste
- Freshly ground black pepper to taste
- ¼ cup chopped cilantro
- 1 ½ cups or 1 can of cooked red kidney beans, rinsed and drained
- ½ small red onion, thinly sliced

Instructions:

1. Put the quinoa and water in small saucepan. Bring the water to a brisk boil and cover the saucepan. Simmer on a low heat until cooked. This would take around 15 minutes or until the quinoa absorbs all the liquid. Remove the saucepan from the heat and let it stand for around 5 minutes.

2. Fluff the quinoa and spread on a flat surface evenly spread to cool and loose the excess liquid. A large dish lined with parchment works best.

3. Finely grate the zest of one orange and set it aside.

4. Segment both of the oranges and squeeze the membranes. The juice yielded will be used later so save it. Save the segments on another side.

5. In a small bowl, whisk together orange zest, 3 tablespoons of orange juice, olive oil, apple cider vinegar, maple syrup, coriander seeds, salt, pepper, and chopped cilantro. Adjust seasonings if desired.

6. Place the orange segments, kidney beans, onion, and quinoa in a large bowl and stir gently to combine.

7. Pour dressing over salad and toss until completely coated.

8. Refrigerate if you are serving later or consume immediately.

Rich Umami French Lentil Salad

Ingredients:

- 1/2 pound (3 cups) dry brown French lentils
- 5 cups vegetable broth (*optional ingredient*)
- 2/3 cup sun-dried tomatoes
- 2 medium red onions
- 2 Bell peppers according to choice of color
- 4 cloves garlic
- 1/2 cup of olive oil, in two places
- 1 cup honey roasted nuts, toasted slightly and roughly chopped. You can choose a mix of your preference
- 1 cup coriander leaves, rustic chopped
- 1 cup mint leaves, rustic chopped
- 1 orange, juiced and zested
- A splash of balsamic vinegar
- 2 tablespoons fresh pomegranate seeds roughly crushed in a mortar to release juices
- Salt according to taste, both for boiling the lentils and adding later
- Black pepper to taste

Instructions:

1. Wash the lentils and put them in a deep saucepan or cooker. Add in the vegetable broth if you are using it or

simply add 5 cups of salted water. Allow to come to a nice boil. Allow the lentils to cook on low flame for around 30 to 40 minutes until they are cooked. Cook them for enough time so that they are tender but are not completely mushy. When they are cooked spread them in an open mouthed container to cool.

2. Finely chop the sun-dried tomatoes and place them in a heat safe container. Pour over the tomatoes around ½ cup of briskly boiling water. Cover and let them steep.

3. Dice the onion.

4. Clean out the bell peppers and dice them.

5. Finely mince the garlic.

6. Heat about 4 tablespoons of olive oil in a sauté pan over medium heat.

7. Add the bell peppers, onion, and the garlic. Cook for about 6-7 minutes. Take off the heat when the onions turn translucent. Make sure not to overcook as we the need the vegetables to be crunchy.

8. Take the tomatoes out of the liquid and reserve around ¼ of the liquid in which they were steeped.

9. In a large bowl mix the lentils with cooked onion mixture. Stir in the tomatoes, the nuts, the chopped coriander and mint as well.

10. In another small bowl mix together the remainder ¼ cup of olive oil, ¼ cup of the steeping liquid, the roughly crushed pomegranate seeds and the orange juice and vinegar.

11. Toss the dressing into the lentils, mix well, and season with pepper and salt according to taste. Enjoy!

Mediterranean Couscous Salad

Ingredients:

- 1 large sweet anise bulb with fronds or celery
- 4tablespoons olive oil, divided
- 1/2 teaspoon ground coriander, toast first and grind; this releases better flavor
- 1 1/2 cups (or 1 15-ounce can) cooked chickpeas, drain any liquid
- 10 Black olives, halved and pitted
- Juice of 1 lemon and its zest
- Juice of 1 orange and its zest
- Salt to taste
- 1 cup couscous (instant version works better)

Instructions:

1. Trim the sweet anise and cut into 1/2 inch thick wedges. Keep the fronds for garnish. (Chop the celery in the same manner if using. Add a teaspoon of fennel seeds.)
2. Heat 2 tablespoons olive oil in a large skillet over a medium heat. Add the sweet anise and cook until tender and caramelized, stirring occasionally. This takes about 12 to 15 minutes.

3. Add the coriander, chickpeas, olives, and lemon juice to the pan and stir to combine. Continue to cook over medium heat, stirring occasionally.

4. Juice the orange into a liquid measuring cup and top off with water to make 2 cups of liquid.

5. Add the liquid to a small saucepan along with 2 tablespoons olive oil, orange zest, lemon zest, and salt. Bring this mixture to a raising boil and stir in couscous. Cover, remove from heat, and let stand for at least 5 minutes.

6. Fluff the couscous grains with a fork and spread out on a serving dish. Spoon the chickpeas and sweet anise over the couscous and garnish with the reserved fronds. Enjoy!

Chapter 13: Desserts

Like mentioned before, desserts on a diet can seem like a quite exiting idea! After all, whenever we think of the word "diet" we always imagine ourselves eating rabbit food and staying away from all desserts. But, these vegan dessert recipes are not only exquisite and heavenly, but also extremely nutritionally rich!

Pear Sorbet

Ingredients:

- 4 kg soft pears, peeled, quartered and cores removed
- 800 ml water
- 800 g caster sugar
- 220 ml grappa, or to taste
- juice and zest of 4 lemons

Instructions:

1. Take a large pan and add the sugar and water to it. Bring the water to a boil and allow it to simmer for 3 minutes.

2. Add the quartered pears to the pan and let it cook for five minutes.

3. Remove the pears from the pan and keep it aside. Add the lemon juice and zest to it.

4. Add the cooked pears to a food processor and blend it well. Transfer the puree to a large dish.

5. Add the grappa to it and mix well.

6. Place the dish in the refrigerator for two hours to allow the sorbet to set. Serve chilled.

Pukka Pineapple with bashed up mint sugar

Ingredients:

- 1 ripe pineapple, peeled and sliced thinly
- 1 handful fresh mint
- natural yoghurt, to serve
- 2 tablespoons caster sugar

Instructions:

1. Arrange the pineapple slices on a large plate.
2. Place the sugar in a mortar. Add the mint leaves to it. Crush the leaves in the mortar and allow the sugar to absorb the mint flavor.
3. Sprinkle the flavored sugar over the pineapple slices.
4. Serve with yogurt.

Mojito Fruit salad

Ingredients:

- 2 ripe pineapples, peeled, cored and cut into chunks
- 2 bunches fresh mint, leaves picked
- ½ large watermelon, peeled and cut into chunks
- 4 tablespoons light brown sugar
- white rum, to taste
- 4 ripe mangoes, stoned and flesh scooped out
- finely grated zest and juice of 6 limes

Instructions:

1. Take a mortar. Add the mint and lime zest to it and grind it.
2. Add the sugar, limejuice and rum to the mint mixture and mix well.
3. Take a large bowl and add all the fruits to it. Pour the Mojito mixture over the fruits and mix well.
4. Garnish the salad with a few mint leaves and serve.

Strawberries with lemon and mint

Ingredients:

- 1600 g strawberries, hulled and quartered
- 8 tablespoons caster sugar
- 16 sprigs mint
- finely grated zest of 4 lemons
- Juice from 4 lemons

Instructions:

1. Take 16 dessert bowls and place them in the freezer to chill. Remove them once they are chilled.
2. Distribute the strawberries evenly among the bowls.
3. Pour the lemon juice on top of the strawberries.
4. Garnish the strawberries with half a tablespoon caster sugar and lemon zest.
5. Top each bowl with a sprig of mint and serve.

Vanilla Ice cream

Ingredients:

- 8 vanilla pods
- 4 teaspoons vanilla-bean paste
- 1200 ml unsweetened soya milk
- 4 x 400 g tin of light coconut milk
- 660 grams agave syrup

Instructions:

1. Take the vanilla pods. Cut them into halves. Add the halves to a large bowl after deseeding them.
2. Pour in the soya milk, coconut milk, vanilla paste and agave syrup. Mix all the ingredients well.
3. Pour the mixture into an ice cream maker. Churn the mixture for around 40 minutes.
4. Pour the churned mixture into a large container.
5. Place the container in the freezer for two hours and allow the ice cream to set. Serve cold.

Easy To Make Vegan Chocolate Cake

Ingredients:
- 3 cups all-purpose flour
- 2 cups white sugar
- 2 teaspoons baking soda
- 1/2 cup cocoa powder
- 1 teaspoon salt
- 2/3 cup oil
- 2 teaspoons distilled white vinegar
- 2 teaspoons vanilla extract
- 2 cups water

Instructions:
1. Crank up your oven to 350 degrees F (175 degrees C) and let it preheat for at least 10 to 20 minutes. Grease a 9 inch baking pan with some vegetable oil or cooking spray.
2. Sieve together the flour, cocoa, salt, sugar and baking soda in a mixing bowl. Pour in the oil, water and distilled white vinegar and mix well until it forms a smooth, lump free batter.
3. Pour the prepared batter into the greased baking dish and pop into the preheated oven.
4. Bake for about 45 minutes or until a skewer inserted in the center of the cake comes out clean.

5. Remove the baking dish from the oven and allow cooling for 5 minutes before inverting the baking dish onto a wire rack. Further cool the cake until it reaches room temperature.

6. Serve with some chocolate sauce and freshly cut strawberries and kiwi.

Vegan Style Banana Muffins

Ingredients:

- 6 cups all-purpose flour
- 2 cups white sugar
- 1 cup brown sugar
- 4 teaspoons ground cinnamon
- 4 teaspoons baking powder
- 2 teaspoons baking soda
- 2 teaspoons ground nutmeg
- 2 teaspoons salt
- 4 cups mashed ripe bananas
- 2 cups canola oil
- 2 cups coconut milk

Instructions:

1. Turn up your oven to 350 degrees F (175 degrees C). Lightly spray a muffin tin with some cooking spray or line with some paper liners. You can even use the reusable silicone muffin molds; just grease them before using.

2. Combine together the white sugar, cinnamon, baking soda, salt, flour, brown sugar, baking powder and nutmeg in a bowl. Add in the mashed bananas, coconut milk and canola oil and mix well to form a smooth, lump free batter.

3. Pour the batter into the prepared muffin tray or muffin molds and pop into the preheated oven. Bake for about 35 to 40 minutes or until a skewer inserted in the center of a muffin comes out clean.

4. Remove the muffin tray or muffin molds from the oven and allow cooling for a few minutes before removing the muffins from the molds.

5. The muffins can be consumed warm or at room temperature, as per preference.

Frozen Avocado, Banana & Chocolate Pudding

Ingredients:

- 2 avocados
- 2 banana
- 2 cups unsweetened soy milk
- 1/2 cup raw cocoa powder
- 1/4 cup agave nectar
- 2 teaspoons lemon juice
- 1/2 cup shredded unsweetened coconut

Instructions:

1. Peel the avocados and remove the pit. Coarsely chop into large chunks. Peel the bananas and coarsely chop them into large chunks.

2. In the jar of the blender, place the avocado and banana chunks and give it a whirl until they get a thick paste like consistency. Slowly pour in the soymilk and blitz again until well combined.

3. Add in the raw cocoa powder, agave nectar, unsweetened coconut and lemon juice into the blender and blend again till it gets a thick consistency.

4. Pour the prepared pudding mix into containers and refrigerate for at least one hour.

5. Serve chilled, topped with some shredded unsweetened coconut.

Delicious Vegan Carrot Cake

Ingredients:

- 1 cup whole wheat flour
- 2 tablespoons soy flour (optional
- 2-1/4 teaspoons ground cinnamon
- 1-1/2 teaspoons ground cloves
- 2 teaspoons baking soda
- 1 teaspoon tapioca starch (optional)
- 1/4 teaspoon salt
- 3/4 cup hot water
- 2 tablespoons flax seed meal
- 1 cup packed brown sugar
- 2 teaspoons vanilla extract
- 6 tablespoons dried currants (optional)
- 3 carrots, grated
- 1/4 cup blanched and slivered almonds (optional)

Instructions:

1. Turn up your oven to 350 degrees F (175 degrees C) and let it preheat for at least 10 to 20 minutes. Grease a 9 inch baking pan with some cooking oil or lightly spray with some cooking spray.

2. Sieve together the whole wheat flour, cinnamon, baking soda, salt, soy flour, ground cloves and tapioca starch in a bowl. Mix well until well combined.

3. In a large mixing bowl, pour the hot water and top with the flax meal. Mix for about a minute until the flax meal starts absorbing the water and the mixture starts to thicken.

4. Add in the vanilla and brown sugar to the flax meal water mix, and keep mixing until the sugar dissolves.

5. Add in the dried currants, blanched and slivered almonds and the grated carrots into the mixture. Mix well to combine.

6. Add the flour mix to the mixing bowl and mix with a light hand. Do not over mix!

7. Pour the prepared batter into the greased baking pan and pop the baking pan into the preheated oven. Bake for about 30 minutes or until a skewer inserted in the center of the cake comes out clean.

8. Remove the pan from the oven and cool for about 10 minutes before inverting the pan onto a wire rack.

9. Cool to room temperature before serving!

Delicious Pumpkin & Tofu Pie

Ingredients:

- ½ cup silken tofu, drained
- 1 cup pumpkin puree
- 6 tablespoons white sugar
- 1/4 teaspoon salt
- 1/2 teaspoon ground cinnamon
- 1/4 teaspoon ground ginger
- 1/8 teaspoon ground cloves
- 1 (5 inch) unbaked pie crust

Instructions:

1. Crank up your oven to 450 degrees F (230 degrees C) and let it preheat for about 10 to 20 minutes.
2. Place the tofu and the pumpkin puree in the jar of the blender. Blend to form a smooth paste. Add the white sugar and blend until the sugar has dissolved.
3. Empty the content of the blender into a mixing bowl. Sprinkle the salt, ground ginger, ground cinnamon and ground cloves into the mixture and mix well.
4. Pour this batter into the unbaked piecrust.
5. Pop into the preheated oven and bake for about 15 minutes. Then, lower the heat to 350 degrees F (175

degrees C), and bake for another 40 minutes more or until a fork inserted in the center of the pie comes out clean.

6. Remove the pie from the oven and let it cool for about 20 minutes before cutting into it.

7. Serve hot or cold, the pie tastes delicious at both temperatures!

Delicious Chocolate Brownies – Vegan Style

Ingredients:

- 1 cup all-purpose flour
- 1 cup white sugar
- 6 tablespoons unsweetened cocoa powder
- 1/2 teaspoon baking powder
- 1/2 teaspoon salt
- 1/2 cup water
- 1/2 cup vegetable oil
- 1/2 teaspoon vanilla extract

Instructions:

1. Crank up your oven to 350 degrees F (175 degrees C) and allow it to preheat for about 10 to 20 minutes. Grease a 9 x 13 inch baking pan with some vegetable oil or spray with some cooking spray.
2. Combine the flour, cocoa powder, salt, sugar and baking powder together in a large bowl. Mix well.
3. Add in the water, vanilla and vegetable oil to the dry ingredients and mix well until the batter gets a smooth, non-lumpy texture.
4. Pour the prepared batter into the greased baking dish and pop into the preheated oven.

5. Let the brownies bake in the preheated oven for about 30 minutes or until the top layer of the brownies stops shining.

6. Remove the baking dish from the oven and allow cooling for about 10 minutes before cutting it into squares.

7. These brownies taste best when they are slightly warm!

Refreshing Lime & Basil Sorbet

Ingredients:

- 1/2 cup sugar
- 1/2 cup water
- 6 tablespoons fresh lime juice
- 10 fresh basil leaves, minced

Instructions:

1. Prepare simple and quick sugar syrup by combining the sugar and water in a small saucepan. Heat the mixture on a medium low flame and let it boil for about one minute, before taking it off heat.

2. While the syrup cools, place the basil leaves in a blender and give them a whirl for a minute, before pouring the lemon juice into the blender jar. Blend for another minute, until it gets a puree like consistency.

3. Once the sugar syrup is at room temperature pour it onto the basil and lemon puree and blend again to combine them together.

4. Pour the prepared mixture into a freezer proof container. Cover with a lid and pop into the freezer for about 3 hours or until the mixture is completely frozen.

5. Spoon out the frozen mixture in small lumps and place in the blender. Blend again until it gets a smooth slushee like texture.

6. Pour the sorbet mix back into the freezer proof container and return to the freezer.

7. If you like big ice crystals in your sorbet, your sorbet is ready to serve, but if you would like smaller crystals, repeat the last two steps a couple more times until you get the desired consistency.

8. Serve chilled, topped with a basil leaf and a thin slice of lime.

Delicious Vegan Style Cheesecake

Ingredients:

- 3 cups soft tofu
- 1 cup soy milk
- 1 cup vegan white sugar
- 2 tablespoons vanilla extract
- 1/2 cup maple syrup
- 2 (9 inch) prepared graham cracker crust
- Sweet berry sauce, to garnish

Instructions:

1. Crank up your oven to 350 degrees F (175 degrees C) and allow it to preheat for at least 10 to 20 minutes.
2. Place the tofu and soymilk in the blender jar together and blitz it until it forms a smooth paste like consistency.
3. Pour the tofu and soy milk mixture into a bowl and add the vegan white sugar to it and mix by hand.
4. Once the sugar has dissolved, add the vanilla extract and maple syrup to it and mix well to combine.
5. Divide the prepared batter between the two graham cracker crusts and pop them into the preheated oven.
6. Bake for about 30 minutes or until a skewer inserted in the center of the cheesecakes comes out clean.

7. Remove the cheesecakes from the oven and cool until it reaches room temperature. Pop the prepared cheesecakes into the refrigerator and chill overnight.

8. Serve chilled, topped with some delicious sweet berry sauce.

Homemade Vegan Marshmallows

Ingredients:

- 1-1/2 cups vegan white sugar

- 2 tablespoons corn syrup

- 1/8 teaspoon salt

- 6 tablespoons water

- 1 teaspoon vanilla extract

- 1/2 cup vegan confectioners' sugar for dusting (if you can't find it, blitz some regular vegan white sugar and run it through a sieve)

Instructions:

1. Spray a 9 x 13 inch baking dish with some cooking spray or grease generously with some oil.

2. Pour the water into a large saucepan. Add the salt, sugar and corn syrup to it and heat on high flame till it reaches 240 degrees F (or 120 degrees C). Drop a little amount of the prepared syrup into a glass of cold water and check if it forms a soft ball. Remove the ball from the water and

place on a flat surface. If the ball collapses on itself and flattens, your syrup is ready. If not, keep heating it.

3. Once the requirement is met, remove the saucepan from heat and using an electric beater, beat the syrup until it forms stiff peaks. This should take about 12 to 15 minutes of beating.

4. Pour in the vanilla extract and mix well using a wooden spoon.

5. Pour the prepared batter into the greased pan and pop the pan into the refrigerator. Chill it overnight or for a minimum of 8 hours.

6. Once set, loosen the edges of the marshmallows using a butter knife. Lightly cover the top of the marshmallows with some confectioner's sugar and invert the tray onto a surface covered with some waxed paper. Dust the other side of the marshmallows with confectioner's sugar again.

7. Cut into bite sized pieces and store in an airtight container.

Oatmeal Flaxseed Cookies

Ingredients:

- 2 cups of rolled oats
- 1 cup brown sugar
- 2/3 cup whole wheat flour
- 2 table spoons of flaxseeds
- 1 tea spoon cinnamon (finely ground)
- 1 tea spoon baking soda
- ½ tea spoon baking powder
- ½ tea spoon salt
- 3/4 cup apple sauce
- 4 table spoons coconut oil
- 1 cup dried cranberries
- ¼ cup shredded unsweetened coconut (optional)

Instructions:

1. Preheat the oven to 350 degrees Fahrenheit (175 degrees Celsius).
2. Prepare a baking sheet by lining it with bakery paper.
3. Mix the oats, flaxseeds, brown sugar, cinnamon, all-purpose flour, baking powder, baking soda, and salt in a bowl. Stir in the applesauce and coconut oil into oat mixture and fold until evenly mixed dough is formed. Next fold in the cranberries into dough. (if using, fold in the

shredded unsweetened coconut at this stage as well)

4. Dollop the dough on to the prepared baking sheet.

5. Bake in the preheated oven until edges of cookies are lightly browned, 10 to 15 minutes.

6. Take them out of the oven and let them cool on a rack. Enjoy the delicious and nutritious cookies as a lovely snack, tea accompaniment or dessert!

Mocha Fudge Bars:

Ingredients:

- 12 ounces of silken tofu (do not drain)
- 2 table spoons canola oil
- 1 pinch salt
- 2 1/3 cup brown sugar
- 1 cup cocoa powder
- 1/3 cup instant coffee powder
- 1 tea spoon vanilla extract
- 1 cup organic whole wheat flour

Instructions:

1. Preheat your oven to 325 degrees Fahrenheit (165 degrees Celsius)

2. Blend tofu until it forms a creamy texture; this can be achieved using an electric blender. Add into it the oil, cocoa, coffee, salt, sugar, and vanilla and mix well until all the ingredients are combined and completely incorporated.

3. Sugar often dissolves last. Make sure it is completely incorporated into the mix and leaves behind no granules. When this stage is reached, remove from the electric blender and manually whisk in the flour. Do this slowly and steadily in order to reduce the chances of any lumps

forming.

4. Pour this batter into a 10x12 inch baking pan; make sure it is greased well with soy margarine.

5. Bake for at least 25 to 30 minutes, or until you can pull the cake away from the sides of the pan without it disintegrating. The mark of this being done is that the bars will have a glossy appearance, which will make them appear slightly underdone.

6. Remove from the oven and allow cooling in the baking pan.

7. Once set, use a clean damp knife to cut out the bars and remove them from the pan. Enjoy these yummy bars as a great pick me up! Chocolate and coffee; nothing can go wrong!

Chocolate and Rum Cheesecake

Ingredients:

- 1 cup of sweet almonds, finely ground
- 1 cup flour (preferentially whole wheat)
- 2/3 cups soy margarine
- 24 ounces of firm tofu
- 1 ½ cups brown sugar
- 7 table spoons of cocoa powder (unsweetened)
- ¼ cup sunflower seed oil
- ½ cup soy milk
- ¼ cup dark rum
- 1 ½ tea spoons vanilla extract

Instructions:

1. Preheat your oven to 325 degrees Fahrenheit (165 degrees Celsius).

2. In a bowl, add the ground almonds and whole wheat flour, mix well to combine. Add in margarine and mix until dough is made.

3. Press the dough into a silicone pan, both on the base and halfway up on the sides. Pan should be around 9 inches.

4. Crumb the tofu in a blender or food processor. Add to the crumbled tofu cocoa, sugar, vanilla, oil, soymilk, and rum. Process until it yields a creamy and smooth mixture. This

makes your filling.

5. Pour this mixture into the set crust.

6. Bake in the preheated oven for approximately 75 minutes, or until filling is set. Let the cake cool on a rack and then place in refrigerator so that it is completely chilled before removing from the pan.

Conclusion

We hope that by now you will have realized that there is more to those humble vegetables and fruits than what meets the eye. Pair the vegan diet with some active exercising and see the change happening within you for yourself.

Veganism is not just a diet; it is a way of life. It is important that you keep an open mind while following this diet. Finding vegan ingredients might take some time, but it is worth all the effort and time that you will put in. At times, you might be tempted to take the easy route and switch over to processed foods and meats, but bear in mind the various benefits of the vegan diet before you yield to the temptation.

The vegan way of life not just aids in weight loss, but also aids in living a healthier lifestyle. When you follow the vegan diet, you consume lesser amounts of artificial components that are often added to the fodder of animals in slaughter houses to increase their size and the yield from them. Very often than not, these artificial components make their way into the meat, milk and eggs of these animals, making them toxic. When you stay off these animal products, you save yourself from these artificial stimulants

We hope that the information provided in this book was inspiring enough to solidify your resolve to be a vegan and aid you in following the vegan way of life without a hitch. Remember, if you think of this as a diet or as a compulsion placed on you, you will never be able to succeed. Rather, think of it as a healthy way of life for a better future. With the change in your perspective towards it, you will find it easier to follow the vegan way of life.

Thank you again for purchasing this book! I wish you a happy and healthy life!

Achieve Your Next Level Health With a Click Away:

Low Carb: Ketogenic Diet to Overcome Belly Fat, Lose Pounds, and Live Healthy

Health and Fitness: Uncommon HIGH Impact Quick Wins You Should Start Today - Nutrition, Natural Health, and Healthy Living

Intermittent Fasting: Shortcut to Build Muscle, Lose Fat, and Easy Weight Loss

Detox: Cleanse for Fast Weight Loss, Anti-Aging, Holistic Healing and Better Health

Other Recommended Books to Become More Effective and Fulfilled In Life:

Self-Improvement: Self Discipline - An Uncommon Guide to Instant Self Control, Incredible Willpower, and Insane Productivity

Spirit Guides: Ultimate Guide to Exploring the Spirit World, Finding Your Angel Guide and Mastering Spirit Communication